Jogging and Walking

For Health and Fitness

Fourth Edition

Frank Rosato, Ed.D.
University of Memphis

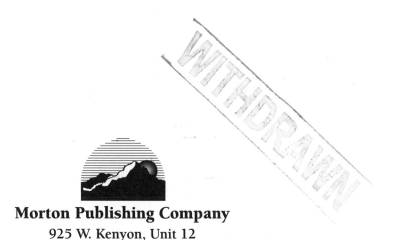

Morton Publishing Company
925 W. Kenyon, Unit 12
Englewood, Colorado 80110

Printed in the United States of America

10 9 8 7 6 5 4 3 2 1

ISBN: 0-89582-546-5

Preface

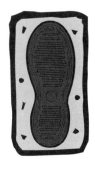

The fields of exercise science and health promotion are dynamic so that the pace of change is accelerating. What was considered to be an article of faith just 5 to 10 years ago may be discarded like a pair of worn out walking or jogging shoes today. In this edition, new information has replaced that which has become outdated, new trends have been identified, and the concepts and content that are presented are supported primarily by research that has been reported since the third edition was published.

The focus of this edition is consistent with that of its predecessors — the emphasis remains on the enhancement of health and fitness. The object is not to take novice exercisers and turn them into fierce competitors although the information in this edition and its intent does not preclude that. But the primary purpose is to take novice exercisers, introduce them to the benefits of walking and jogging, and present persuasive and logical reasons why they should take the time and make the effort to include exercise in their daily lives. The emphasis is to encourage ordinary Americans to start moving for health enhancement, or for improvement in physical appearance, or for the development of physical fitness, or for other reasons.

This edition provides the guidelines for novices to begin and sustain a walking or jogging program safely and effectively. The principles of exercise are presented, which appropriately applied by walkers and joggers, will result in the accomplishment of their health and fitness objectives. Also, veteran walkers and joggers may find information that is useful both for motivation and for refining established programs.

Nutrition is an important component of a healthy lifestyle and certainly important for active people. The latest nutritional concepts — the Food Guide Pyramid, new food labels for processed items, the antioxidant vitamins, phytochemicals, etc. — are presented. The consistent application of sound nutritional concepts is beneficial to walkers and joggers as they attempt to achieve their objectives.

Guidelines and precautions for exercise in hot and cold weather are covered. Understanding the challenges imposed by both is the key to exercising effectively and safely in various environmental conditions. The prevention and treatment of common walking and running injuries are covered.

Finally, this edition is accompanied by an instructor's manual that should facilitate the preparation, delivery, and assessment of instructional and learning objectives. The Instructor's Manual includes learning objectives, chapter outlines (lecture outlines), and a test bank, consisting of true-false, multiple choice, definition, and short essay items. There are more than 500 test questions available for instructors to use in constructing their tests. The Instructor's Manual will be made available to adopters of the book.

I would like to thank the staff at Morton Publishing Company for their patience and flexibility associated with deadlines as I prepared the manuscript. Special thanks to Devonia Cage who, after putting in her regular day at work, took my handwritten manuscript home where she quickly turned it into a computer driven hard copy. Finally, I would like to thank my wife Pat for her patience and willingness to take on some of my home responsibilities while I was involved in this project.

Frank Rosato, Ed.D.
University of Memphis

Contents

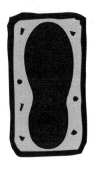

Physical Fitness: An Overview

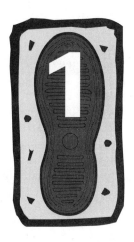

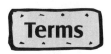

Body composition
Cardiorespiratory endurance
Cardiovascular diseases
Chronic diseases
Communicable diseases
Coronary heart disease
Degenerative diseases
Flexibility
Health-related fitness
Muscular endurance
Muscular strength
Performance-related fitness
Risk factor

National polls and surveys and the mass media have documented the extent of the physical fitness movement in the United States highlighting the segments of society that are heavily involved as well as those who are conspicuous by their absence. This chapter includes the latest exercise guidelines developed by the American College of Sports Medicine (ACSM) and the Centers for Disease Control and Prevention (CDC), along with their rationales.

Fitness and wellness programs in the workplace have existed long enough to reach preliminary conclusions about their cost-effectiveness. These early data are encouraging in light of health-care costs. The average workweek has expanded in the last 15 years while the hours available for leisure time have declined. People are having trouble finding time for exercise. Therefore, time management skills and techniques are taking on more importance. Some time management tools are presented here to help people find pockets of time during the day for worthwhile pursuits such as exercise. Finally, a rationale is included for choosing walking/ jogging as a safe and expeditious mode of activity for attaining physical fitness and health enhancement.

AMERICA ON THE MOVE

Throughout the United States, we see people walking, jogging, cycling, and swimming to attain physical fitness, weight loss, and other health-promoting reasons. Fitness clubs are packed with people doing aerobics to music and exercising with weights, stair-steppers, rowing machines, treadmills, and bikes. Exercise equipment is becoming more and more sophisticated every day. Information regarding fitness and health appear in the print and electronic media daily.

From this frenzy of activity, the perception easily could be that most Americans are fully involved in the exercise movement. Unfortunately, perception and reality are not in agreement. Information gathered during the last 30 years indicates that most Americans have not exercised enough to have a positive impact on their fitness level or their health status. Data accumulated on U. S. adults over the past couple of decades indicate that:[1]

1. 15% participate regularly (three times per week for at least 30 minutes) in vigorous physical activities that are not work-related

2. 22% participate regularly (five times per week for at least 30 minutes) in sustained physical activity during nonworking hours

3. 25% engage in no physical activity during nonworking hours

4. More than 60% engage in no exercise or participate sporadically or marginally so no improvement in health status results

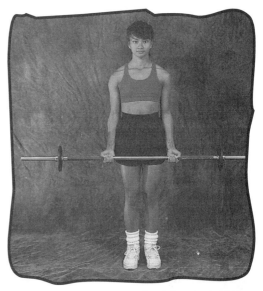

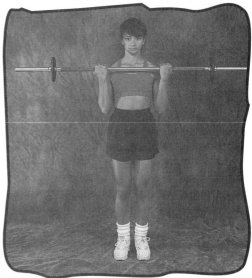

Exercise equipment is becoming more sophisticated.

Exercising with free weights is increasingly popular with women.

5. Only half of young people (12 to 21 years of age) participate regularly in vigorous physical activity

6. One-fourth of young people (12 to 21 years of age) report no participation at all.

The current trend toward exercise began in the 1960s. During the early years, literally millions of sedentary people began exercising and the movement grew rapidly. Eventually the influx of new participants slowed. In the past few years a disturbing trend has begun to surface: The exercise movement has plateaued in spite of growth in the population.[2] This is occurring at a time when the health and wellness benefits associated with consistent participation in physical activities is most compelling.

The American Heart Association (AHA) has recognized the importance of physical activity by declaring in 1992 that its opposite, physical inactivity, is a major risk for **cardiovascular disease**.[3] Further, the AHA stated, "Persons of all ages should include physical activity in a comprehensive program of health promotion and disease prevention."[4] In 1985, The American Cancer Society began recommending exercise to help people protect themselves from cancer.[5] The endorsements of exercise by such prestigious organizations came about because of the weight of research evidence.

SURVEY RESULTS

A compilation of data by the authors of the *Surgeon General's Report on Physical Activity and Health* in 1996 indicated that the most popular leisure-time physical activity by far was walking, followed by gardening or yardwork, stretching exercises, cycling, strength building exercises, stair climbing, jogging, aerobics, and swimming.[6]

Another analysis of fitness participation and fitness equipment use that examined the period from 1987 to 1997 in the United States revealed several trends:[7]

1. 63% more people used cardiorespiratory equipment, and 44% more used strength-training equipment in 1997 than in 1987.

2. Weight-training use of free weights (barbells and dumbbells) rose from 24.5 million in 1987 to 43.2 million in 1997; 39% of free-weight users were women.

3. The popularity of treadmills for walking and jogging increased by 720% in that time period.

4. Membership in health clubs increased by 63%.

5. Purchases of fitness equipment for the home skyrocketed; nearly one-third of all households bought and used exercise equipment during the 10-year period.

6. Baby boomers (now entering their 50s) remain committed to exercise.

7. Participation in high-impact and step aerobics declined, and group exercise classes increased, as did low-impact activities such as yoga; exercise equipment became more innovative and diversified in an effort to cater to exercise interests.

8. The popularity of personal trainers increased significantly. An estimated 15,000 aspiring exercise professionals took the personal trainer certification exam in 1998 — up from 3,367 in 1992.

A study by the National Sporting Goods Association (NSGA) indicated an increase in exercise participation by older Americans.[8] Participation in seven fitness activities by the 75-and-older age group increased by 27%. Participation by the 55-to-64 age group in these activities increased by 17%. Contrast that to a 4% drop in participation in the 25-to-34 age group. The seven fitness activities in the study were aerobic exercise, cycling, calisthenics, exercise with equipment, exercise walking, jogging and swimming.

According to NSGA, 20.4 million women claim to be exercisers, compared to 15.5 million men, and 23% of the women exercise regularly, compared to 19% for men.[9] Frequency of exercise was defined as participating in physical activity at least twice a week. Two times per week is not enough of an exercise stimulus to improve health significantly, and it is below the American College of Sports Medicine's recommendation for frequency of exercise.

Although the data on the increasing number of older people who exercise is encouraging, the decline in exercise participation for both males and females as they age indicates that, on the whole, this age group exercises less than all other age groups.[10] People who exercise vigorously and frequently are primarily young adults in the middle and upper socioeconomic strata of U.S. society as defined by income, education, and occupation. In general, professionals are more active than blue-collar workers in their leisure time. Blue-collar workers as a group, however, particularly those with fewer than 12 years of education, report more on-the-job physical activity than do professionals.[11] The lower intensity on-the-job expenditure of energy over a 7- to 8-hour day tends to equalize the energy expended by those who participate in structured exercises of higher intensity for 45 to 60 minutes four to five times per week.

The exercise movement that began in the late 1960s grew rapidly during the 1970s and continued through the mid-1980s, at which point it slowed down and finally plateaued during the 1990s. Annual surveys conducted by Louis Harris and Associates show that the percentage of Americans who exercise strenuously has not changed significantly during the last 10 years or so.[12] Strenuous exercise was defined as breathing heavily with heart rate and pulse rate accelerated for at least 20 minutes, at least 3 days per week. In spite of the media hype, studies show that today's fitness movement is flat and the majority of Americans are not exercising. One of the many consequences of a sedentary lifestyle is the rising rate of overweight and obesity. Current estimates indicate that 55%, or 97 million people in the United States, are overweight.[13]

Although physical inactivity is a **risk factor** that crosses all demographic boundaries, the problem is worse for: (a) minority ethnic groups, (b) all people regardless of their ethnicity who are poorly educated, (c) older adults, and (d) those of lower socioeconomic status. Unfortunately, **chronic diseases** such as heart disease, stroke, diabetes, and obesity — all of which respond positively to regular exercise — are most prevalent in these population groups.

Physical inactivity is a risk factor that can be reversed easily and economically. The new recommendation for exercise developed jointly by the American College of Sports Medicine and the Centers for Disease Control and Prevention for the purpose of health enhancement is that adults should accumulate at least 30 minutes of moderate physical activity over the course of most days (at least 4 days per week).[14] Scientific research has indicated quite clearly that compliance with this modest level of exercise can improve the health of individuals and, concomitantly, the health of the nation.

Furthermore, exercise does not have to be structured or planned, nor must it include the activities associated most with fitness and health — jogging, cycling, rowing, swimming, and the like. Although vigorous exercises such as these provide the most benefit, more moderate exercises including, but not limited to, everyday physical activities such as mowing the lawn (without a riding mower), gardening, raking leaves, walking, climbing stairs, and washing and waxing the car contribute to better health. In addition, exercise in a single continuous session is not necessary.

A total of 30 minutes of physical activities broken up into three 10-minute bouts is just as effective as one continuous bout for health enhancement. All activities that require some amount of physical exertion should be approached as opportunities for exercise and a bonus for health enhancement even if they must be sprinkled throughout the day. Intermittent low-intensity physical activity spread throughout the day might not improve one's level of physical fitness measurably, but it nevertheless does burn calories. For example, an office worker who spends 2 minutes an hour to send e-mail to co-workers day after day instead of walking down the hall to speak to them personally would gain the energy equivalent of 11 pounds of fat over a decade. This is a substantial weight gain over time from a tiny amount of energy saved.[15]

Add this to all of the other ways at our disposal for saving energy, and we can easily see that the problem becomes compounded; in 10 years the weight gain is 30 pounds instead of 11. A Scottish researcher estimates that labor-saving devices that affect home life, recreation, and occupation have reduced average energy expenditures in the United Kingdom by 800 calories per day over the last 25 years.[16]

We all can benefit by adopting the philosophy that substituting our own muscle power for mechanically and electronically powered devices is an idea whose time is well past due. When possible, we should walk or bike instead of driving the car, climb stairs instead of using elevators and escalators, take a 10-minute walk instead of a cup of coffee and a doughnut at breaktime, mow our own lawn instead of hiring someone else to do it, and wash our own car instead of running it through the car wash. By taking advantage of these and many other opportunities for physical activity, a person surely will meet the minimum criteria for health enhancement and will look better and feel better as a result.

The first two editions of this text were concerned with jogging as the means for attaining fitness and health. The third and fourth editions of the text have been expanded by the addition of walking, to reflect the new guidelines for and attitude toward exercise. In Chapters 5 and 6 you will be introduced to the benefits of walking for health.

EXERCISE PROGRAMS IN BUSINESS AND INDUSTRY

Data that are accumulating from worksite exercise programs have provided more ammunition for the physically active life. Many of these programs have been in place long enough to have had an impact on employee health. As they attempt to contain the spiraling cost of health care, companies that have invested in worksite health-promotion programs are saving more dollars than they spent initially.

For preventive practices to translate into changes in health status it takes time and consistent effort. An educational component is necessary to change longstanding behavior patterns such as cigarette smoking, poor nutritional practices, and sedentary living. Time and a sincere commitment are required to control blood pressure and serum levels of cholesterol with lifestyle changes instead of medications.

Early data coming from worksite health-promotion programs are encouraging. Companies are discovering that health-care costs are lower, worker absenteeism is down, employee productivity is up, and on-the-job accidents are fewer.[17] Health-promotion programs with physical fitness opportunities either on-site or paid for (partially or fully) by the company are perks to recruit and keep key personnel.

The worksite has great potential for adults to engage in regular physical exercise. In fact, the goals established for worksite fitness programs in *Healthy People 2000* — a national study in which thousands of health professionals contributed to the development of specific national objectives — were exceeded. The more recent *Healthy People 2010* objectives have set worksite fitness goals higher with the expectation that these, too, will be met and exceeded.[18]

The cost of operating a worksite physical fitness program usually can be recovered within a few years. The economic benefits that accrue from quality fitness programs surpass the costs to the company. The latter costs include, among others, professional leadership, facilities, equipment, marketing, and promotion.[19]

THE COSTS OF SEDENTARY LIVING

Exercise of moderate intensity, performed consistently, reduces all-cause mortality, increases longevity, and delays or reduces the likelihood of incurring chronic diseases.[20] The most active and most physically fit people have death rates from all causes that are 25% to 50% lower than those who are least active or least fit.[21] A low level of fitness is one of the most potent risk factors for death from all causes in males, and it is at least as risky as smoking cigarettes.[22] Many of the deaths associated with physical inactivity are premature. The number of lives lost because of inactivity is approximately 200,000 a year.[23] When inactivity is combined with a poor diet, the annual death rate increases to about 300,000.

Exercising regularly also delays or reduces the likelihood of succumbing to one or more of the chronic diseases. As a result, active people place less demand on the nation's medical delivery system, and they are more productive occupationally. Conversely, those who choose to lead sedentary lives impose the costs associated with their lifestyle on others.

The financial cost to others (referred to as "external costs") by those who are physically inactive result from payments they receive from collectively financed programs such as health insurance, sick-leave payments, disability insurance, and group life insurance. To finance these programs, active people pay the same premiums and payroll taxes as the sedentary people who are the most frequent users. These programs do not distinguish frequency of utilization nor do they provide discounts for positive health behaviors; therefore, they essentially function as social welfare programs that subsidize unhealthy behaviors.

When sedentary people gravitate to an active way of life, everyone benefits. Each minute that people spend walking increases life expectancy by one minute.[24] Because joggers burn calories twice as fast as non-joggers, the former can expect a return of double their exercise time in life expectancy. The Rand Corporation, a well-known California based "think tank," has developed a theoretical model that projects the following: Each mile that a sedentary person walks or jogs will add 21 minutes to that person's life and save society 24 cents in medical and other costs.[25] The economic drain of sedentary living on society is double the external cost associated with cigarette smoking.

CONTRIBUTING TO THE PROBLEM

The fitness movement developed largely as a reaction to innovations in medicine, science, and technology and their relationship to the changing patterns of disease and death patterns in the United States. **Communicable diseases** (tuberculosis, pneumonia, typhoid fever, smallpox, scarlet fever, and others) were the leading causes of death during the early years of the 20th century.

Advances in medical science have virtually eradicated these maladies and threats to life, but they have been replaced by chronic **degenerative diseases** such as heart disease, stroke, cancer, diabetes, and the like. This group of diseases is largely lifestyle-induced and has reached epidemic proportions. Many authorities refer to these diseases as voluntary or self-inflicted, thereby emphasizing the influence of negative choices and unhealthy behaviors on the development and course of these diseases.

Cardiovascular diseases accounts for approximately 42% of all deaths in the United States.[26] Approximately 57,490,000 people in the United States have one or more forms of cardiovascular disease.[27] Cardiovascular diseases are responsible for 950,000 deaths annually, and about half of these (500,000) are the result of **coronary heart disease**. Although most Americans are aware of this type of heart disease, most people don't fully understand the behaviors necessary to prevent or delay it. The Framingham Heart Study — a landmark study of heart disease — identified the risk factors connected with heart disease. This ongoing study began in 1949 and continues to this day turning out valuable information from the subjects they began studying decades ago.

As risk factors were identified, the realization evolved that heart disease was not the inevitable consequence of aging but, instead, an acquired disease that is potentially preventable. Cigarette smoking, high blood pressure, elevated levels of blood fats, diabetes, overweight, stress, lack of exercise, and a family history of heart disease were found to be highly related to heart attack and stroke. Most of these risk factors can be modified by the way we live.

Within our control are opportunities to choose what to eat and how much, whether to smoke cigarettes, whether to exercise, and how to control stress. We can choose when to be screened for blood pressure and blood fats, and we can choose whether to act upon that information. During the last four decades, millions of Americans have changed eating, smoking, and exercise habits. Consequently, deaths from cardiovascular disease declined by approximately 51% during this time.[28] Even though other factors are involved in this favorable trend, modifications in lifestyle have made a significant contribution.

Our lives today are considerably different from life in the early years of this century. Scientific and technological advances have made us functionally mechanized. Labor-saving devices proliferate in all phases of life — occupation, home life, and leisure-time pursuits — always with the promise of more and better to come. Each new invention, helped foster a receptive attitude toward a life of ease, and we have become accustomed to the easy way of doing things. The mechanized way is usually the most expedient way, and in our time-oriented society, this became another stimulus to indulge in the sedentary life.

Today, exercise for fitness is programmed into our lives as an entity separate from our other functions. In contrast, the energy expenditures of our forebears were integrated into their work, play, and home life. Physical fitness was necessary, and fit people were the rule rather than the exception. Tilling the soil, digging ditches, and working in factories were physically demanding jobs. Lumberjack contests and square dances were vigorous leisure pursuits. Being a wife and taking care of home and family required long hours doing arduous tasks. In the early years of this century, one-third of the energy for operating factories came from muscle power. By 1970, this figure had dropped to less than 1%, reflecting the declining energy demand of our jobs.

The turn of the century found 70% of the population working long, hard hours to produce food. Children of this era walked several miles to school and did chores when they returned home. Today, only 3% of the population, using highly mechanized equipment, are involved in the production of food, and their children ride in motor vehicles to school. Adults drive to the store, circle the parking lot to get as close as possible to the entrance, and ride elevators and escalators while there. We mow the lawn with a riding mower, play golf in a cart, wash dishes and clothes in appropriate appliances, change television channels with a remote control, and open garage doors in the same manner.

These are simply observations of life in the United States. This is not to imply that the fruits of science and technology should be repudiated but, rather, that the results, along with their impact upon us, be viewed in perspective and acted upon accordingly. Inventions of the industrial age have significantly reduced the level of physical activity required to earn a living. Machines and automation have taken much of the physical labor out of our occupations. The effect has ramifications from farm to factory. Home life and leisure pursuits have been affected as well. And now we find ourselves moving at the speed of light into the "information age," with its potential for further reducing the need for physical activity. Cell phones, faxes, electronic mail, and the proliferation of computers for business and home have changed the way we do business and access information — and all of this is accomplished while we sit down.[29]

The leisure-time activities of young people 10 to 17 years of age also have changed. Computerized games, video games, and television watching have replaced more active leisure-time games and activities. These sedentary pursuits seem to be contributing to the rise in obesity occurring in this age group in the United States today. At least one study has shown that the metabolic rate (the rate at which the body burns calories) of children was lower while watching television than it was during a comparable period of rest.[30] Reducing TV viewing time by just 3 hours per week and converting those hours to moderately intense physical activity would improve physical fitness and health status for this age group.

Futurists of the 1960s predicted that technology would take over many of the laborious tasks in the workplace as well as the home. The result of all of this would be a substantial reduction in the time required to earn a living and to manage the household, leaving us with an abundance of free time. Obviously this prediction was off the mark and has not materialized for much of the population. At that time, the expectation was that the new technology would enable the workforce to do the work in less time, and this ultimately would lead to a 4-day workweek.

In reality, the new technology enabled U.S. workers to do more work in the same amount of time, thereby increasing productivity with less energy expended. As corporations have downsized, fewer workers using modern technology and working longer hours are more productive than the full workforce used to be.

This trend has increased the difficulty of finding time to schedule exercise. Effective management of time is becoming more important as we attempt to balance work, leisure activity, and sleep in a 24-hour day. To commit the time and effort required to exercise consistently, we must understand its relevance to a healthy life.

MANAGING TIME

Effective time managers are skilled in identifying and prioritizing goals. They identify the ultimate objective and then set realistic short-term goals that are attainable with sustained effort. The goals that are established should be specific so progress can be evaluated. Finally, goals should be accompanied by a timeline for accomplishments.

Wise time managers use a variety of tools to help them accomplish their daily tasks. For example, many people generate a list of things to do for that day. They carry the list with them on a 3 x 5 index card or pocket-size notebook and cross off the tasks as they are completed during the day.

Another useful tool is a weekly or monthly calendar. The calendar contains the fixed items that occur every week, such as classes, work, meals, and meetings. Also included are important non-fixed items such as tests, due dates for written and oral assignments, and vacation. Filling out a calendar like this indicates pockets of time available for physical activity, study, and other pursuits. When total time is examined systematically, you would be surprised how much time is left over.

As important as time availability is, individuals still must be motivated to use it constructively. A national survey conducted among "less active" Americans indicated that 84% watched television a minimum of 3 hours per week.[31] This suggests that they have leisure time available but would rather watch television than participate in physical activity. Television viewing is running into stiff competition from another sedentary pursuit — the home computer — and this is compounding the difficulty of finding time for physical pursuits.

RATIONALE FOR CHOOSING WALKING AND JOGGING

Although people have inhabited the earth for many centuries, only during the last 75 years have such drastic changes in lifestyle been generated. Our basic need for physical activity has not changed. Our bodies were constructed for, and thrive on, physical work, but we find ourselves thrust into the automobile, television, and sofa age, and we simply have not had enough time to adapt to this new sedentary way of living. Perhaps 100,000 years from now, the sedentary life will be the healthy life. At this stage of our development, though, the law of use and disuse continues to work: That which is used becomes stronger, and that which is not used becomes weaker. For simple verification of this physiological principle, witness the results of a leg in a cast for 8 weeks and note the atrophy of the limb that has occurred during that time.

Many people, myself included, believe that our new ways of living are precipitating, or at least significantly contributing to, the diseases that are affecting modern affluent humankind. These ways of living are unique to highly industrialized nations. By contrast, the underdeveloped nations, with their different lifestyles, do not experience this phenomenon to the same extent.

Before developing or engaging in any form of physical exercise program, beginners should determine what their expectations are. What goals, both short- and long-term do you wish to achieve? Identifying goals will guide you regarding how hard, how often, how long, and what activities will comprise your exercise program. Once you resolve these questions, you can tailor the program to meet your specific objectives. If you follow through, you will have a high probability of success.

The choice to walk, jog, or to combine the two as the activity mode by which to attain health and fitness objectives has a significant base of support in research. Both activities are effective and popular.

Walking

For human beings, walking is the natural form of locomotion. It is a low-risk, low-impact activity that can be done almost anywhere, by almost anybody (including many who have disabilities), in most environments, and within a reasonable timeframe.

Walking uses a heel-to-toe motion so the foot strike at landing is at the heel and the push-off is at the end of the big toe. This action dissipates the force of impact with the ground over

Identifying goals will guide you regarding how hard, how often, how long, and what activities will comprise your exercise program.

the widest possible foot area. The foot rolling forward generates horizontal momentum for forward movement. The advancing foot lands before the rear foot leaves the ground, ensuring that one foot is always in contact with the ground. Forward motion of this type minimizes the impact of landing.

For beginners, walking is an effective introduction to physical activity. Walking can be manipulated to meet a variety of objectives. In addition to being an entry point into exercise, it can be a lead-up conditioner for other types of activity. Or it can be the end product for developing and maintaining physical fitness. This can be accomplished through brisk walking, or variations such as speed walking, power walking, and race walking.

Millions of people are walking for health and fitness. More than 10,000 walking events are held annually. These include walk-a-thons, fun walks, and competitive race walks. More than 6,500 walking clubs are scattered throughout the country. Some of these feature hiking and orienteering (using a map and compass to find the path between two land marks).

Slow walking speeds produce substantial health benefits but result in a minimal increase in fitness level. Higher speeds result in improvements in both health and fitness. In one study, women subjects were divided into three groups of different walking intensity.[32] One group walked at 3 miles per hour (mph) (strollers), a second group walked at 4 mph (brisk walkers), and the last group walked at 5 mph (aerobic walkers). The subjects walked 3 miles per day, 5 days per week. At the end of 24 weeks, the data were analyzed. The results indicated that physical fitness improved on a dose-response basis — that is, the fastest walking group improved the most, and the slowest walking group improved the least. The risk of cardiovascular disease was reduced equally among the three groups. The 3 mph walkers benefited as much as the fastest walkers with regard to favorably changing the cardiovascular risk profile. If enhancement of health is the major exercise objective, walking — even slow walking — fits the bill nicely. If, however, the major objective is to improve physical fitness, fast walking is a satisfactory activity. The bonus for those who engage in exercise for the purpose of fitness is that they achieve the health benefits simultaneously.

Jogging

Jogging is a higher impact activity than walking. Jogging requires that both feet must be off the ground for a split-second during every stride. Because joggers become airborne, their impact with the ground is greater and the expenditure of energy is higher than that of walking except under two circumstances.

1. The energy expenditure or oxygen cost of very slow jogging (5 mph) is equal to walking at the same speed. At speeds faster than 5 mph, the oxygen cost of walking exceeds that of jogging because of the inefficiency associated with very fast walking.

2. The oxygen cost of jogging up a hill is about half that of walking up the same hill. Both feet come off the ground during jogging, so some of the vertical lift needed to run up the hill occurs naturally, thereby lowering the net cost of the vertical work.

Some surfaces are better than others. Still, jogging can be pursued almost anywhere that is devoid of hazards such as potholes or jutting rocks. It also is time-effective. For instance, a person might take 1 hour to walk 4 miles but only 35 to 40 minutes to slow-jog the same distance. The savings in time is important to many busy people.

Even though the popularity of jogging has declined somewhat in the last few years, it nonetheless remains alive and kicking. An estimated 20 million people jog a minimum of three times per week.[33] Studies have shown that joggers are highly dedicated to this activity and are compliant exercisers. Jogging will remain an effective means of improving health and fitness and likely will continue to appeal to a large number of participants.

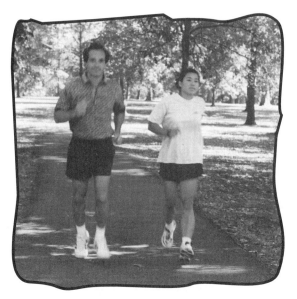

A person can walk or jog alone . . .
or with someone else.

Other factors contribute to the appeal of walking and jogging, too. These activities can be done either indoors or outdoors and in most environmental conditions. From the perspective of clothing and equipment needs, a good pair of shoes is mandatory for protection against potential injury. The environmental conditions should dictate the remainder of the attire.

Another appealing factor is that participants can walk or jog alone or with others. Walking or jogging in solitude provides the opportunity for introspection, or to mentally organize that paper that you have to write for class, or it provides a setting for the mind to roam freely. Walking or jogging also provides the opportunity for socialization and camaraderie with friends who are interested in the same form of exercise, and it is an ideal circumstance for conversation.

HEALTH-RELATED FITNESS

The primary purposes of health-related exercise are the prevention of disease and the attainment of well-being. This can be achieved by consistent participation in mild to moderately vigorous aerobic activities. The components of **health-related fitness** are (1) **cardiorespiratory endurance,** which is the maximum ability to take in, deliver, and extract oxygen for physical work, (2) **muscular strength,** which is the maximum amount of force that a muscle or group of muscles can exert in a single contraction, (3) **muscle endurance,** which is the capacity to exert repetitive muscular force, (4) **flexibility,** which is the range of movement around the joints of the body, and (5) **body composition,** which is the amount of fat versus lean tissue in the body. Figure 1.1 illustrates the components of health-related fitness.

Attaining aerobic physical fitness requires individuals to exercise vigorously enough to improve their cardiorespiratory endurance and muscle endurance. Exercises for the development and maintenance of physical fitness increase the energy level and enhance physical appearance. A standard for aerobic fitness is exercise 5 days per week, for approximately 45 minutes per exercise session, at an intensity level of 70% to 80% of the maximum heart rate (discussed in Chapter 3).

PERFORMANCE-RELATED FITNESS

Performance-related fitness requires the abilities necessary for proficient execution of sports skills. Although these abilities are not necessary to enhance health, they are indispensable to those who participate competitively in physical activities. The performance-related components are speed, power, balance, coordination, agility, and reaction time. Successful performance in games such as racquetball, tennis, basketball, volleyball, and badminton — to name a few — is dependent upon these athletic abilities. The

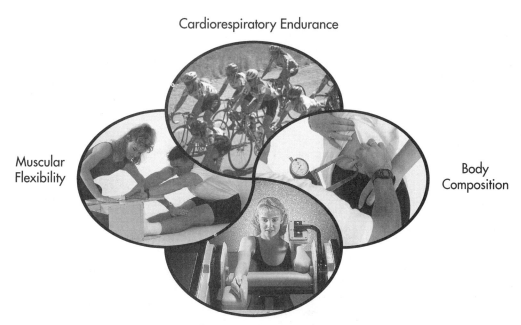

Cardiorespiratory Endurance

Muscular Flexibility

Body Composition

Muscular Strength and Endurance

Figure 1.1 Health-related components of physical fitness.

health-related and performance-related components are not mutually exclusive. Some individuals perform in athletic contests as a means by which to meet their health-related goals. A competitor in an endurance event is developing health-related components even though the major goal is performance-related. A perceived lack of athletic ability should not be a barrier to exercise for health enhancement because many health-related activities require little athletic ability. Walking and jogging are prime examples.

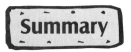

Summary

- Most people in the United States do not exercise often enough or vigorously enough to improve their health.

- The exercise movement has plateaued in the last few years despite compelling evidence that exercise is necessary for health and wellness.

- Mechanization, the product of science and technology, has removed much of the labor from our occupations, homes, and leisure time activities.

- The American Heart Association has classified physical inactivity as a major risk factor for heart disease.

- Less than one-fourth of adults in the United States are exercising at the level recommended for heart health.

- Physical inactivity is more prevalent among (a) minority groups, (b) poorly educated people, (c) older adults, and (d) those who are in the lower socioeconomic levels.

- For health enhancement, the American College of Sports Medicine recommends participation in mild to moderate physical activity for at least 30 minutes 4 days a week.

- Everyday activities such as walking, climbing stairs, mowing the lawn, raking leaves, and similar activities contribute to health.

- A person doesn't have to exercise in one continuous bout; it can be done at various times during the day.

- Fitness and wellness worksite programs are cutting the cost of health care as a result of less absenteeism, greater productivity and fewer on-the-job accidents.

- Consistent participation in exercise reduces the risk of mortality from all causes.

- People who have a sedentary lifestyle receive more payments from health insurance, disability insurance, and group life insurance, and take more sick leave than physically active people.

- The Rand Corporation has estimated that each mile a sedentary person walks or jogs will add 21 minutes to that person's life and save society 24¢ in medical and other costs.

- Risk factors for heart disease, identified by researchers who participated in the Framingham Study, are cigarette smoking, high blood pressure and blood fats, diabetes, overweight, stress, lack of exercise, and a family history of heart disease.

- The death rate from cardiovascular disease has declined by more than 50% in the last four decades.

- The workweek has been on the increase during the decades of the 1980s and 1990s.

- As leisure time decreases, time-management skills assume greater importance as we attempt to balance work and play. Time management techniques are available to help us organize our time.

- Walking for exercise is a low-risk, low-impact activity that can be done in most environments and can satisfy the needs of beginners and experienced exercisers alike.

- Walking can enhance health and develop aerobic fitness.

- Jogging is a higher impact activity than walking; it uses more energy and requires more oxygen under most conditions.

- ◆ At approximately 5 mph, the oxygen cost of walking is equal to that of jogging.

- ◆ Walking up hills requires more oxygen than jogging up the same hills.

- ◆ Walking and jogging can be done indoors or outdoors.

- ◆ A quality pair of shoes is the only equipment or special clothing necessary for walkers and joggers.

- ◆ Walking and jogging contribute to the health-related fitness components: cardiorespiratory endurance, muscular strength and endurance, flexibility, and body composition.

- ◆ The components of performance-related fitness are speed, power, coordination, agility, balance, and reaction time.

1. National Center for Chronic Disease Prevention and Health Promotion, *Physical Activity and Health: A Report of the Surgeon General*, (Atlanta: Centers for Disease Control and Prevention, 1996).
2. Ibid.
3. "It's Official: Inactivity Increases Coronary Risks," *Harvard Health Letter*, 3:3 (1992), 8.
4. "It's Official: Inactivity Increases Coronary Risks."
5. *Cancer Facts and Figures 1992* (Atlanta: American Cancer Society, 1997).
6. CDC, *Physical Activity and Health*.
7. *Tracking the Fitness Movement, 1987–1997: A Decade of Change* (North Palm Beach, FL: Fitness Products Council, 1998).
8. "Older Adults and Women Exercise the Most," *Fitness Management*, 14:11 (Oct. 1998), 8–10.
9. Ibid.
10. D. C. Nieman, *Exercise Testing and Prescription A Health-Related Approach* (Mountain View, CA: Mayfield, 1999).

11. P. C. Wagener, *Health Conditions Among the Currently Employed: United States, 1988* (National Center for Health Statistics, Series 10, No. 186 (PHS) 93-1412) (Washington, DC: U. S. Government Printing Office, 1993).
12. T. Dybdahl, *The Prevention Index '97: A Report Card on the Nation's Health* (Emmaus, PA: Rodale Press, 1997).
13. "Majority of Americans Considered Overweight," *Fitness Management*, 14:11 (Oct. 1998), 14.
14. R. R. Pate, M. Pratt, S. N. Blair, et al. "Physical Activity and Public Health: A Recommendation from the Centers for Disease Control and Prevention and the American College of Sports Medicine," *Journal of the American Medical Association*, 273 (1995), 402–407.
15. B. Liebman, "Take a Hike" Interview with Steve Blair, *Nutrition Action Healthletter*, 26:1 (Jan./Feb., 1999), 1–7.
16. Ibid.
17. U. S. Dept. of Health and Human Services, *Healthy People 2010 Objectives* (Washington, DC: U. S. Government Printing Office, 1998).
18. Ibid.

19. J. C. Erfurt, A. Foote, M. A. Heirich, and B. M. Rock, *The Wellness Outreach at Work Program: A Step-by-Step Guide*, (NIH Publication No. 95–3043) (Washington DC: National Institute of Health, Aug. 1995).
20. Erfurt et al.; S. N. Blair, J. B. Kampert, H. W. Kohl, et al., "Influences of Cardiorespiratory Fitness and Other Resources on Cardiovascular Disease and All-Cause Mortality in Men and Women," *Journal of the American Medical Association*, 276 (1996): 205–210; S. N. Blair, H. W. Kohl, C. E. Barlow et al., "Changes in Physical Fitness and All-Cause Mortality: A Prospective Study of Healthy and Unhealthy Men," *Journal of the American Medical Association*, 273 (1995): 1093–1098; I. M. Lee and R. S. Paffenbarger, "Do Physical Activity and Physical Fitness Avert Premature Mortality?" *Exercise and Sport Science Reviews*, 24 (1996): 135–169; L. H. Kushi, R. M. Fee, and A. R. Folsom et al., "Physical Activity and Mortality in Postmenopausal Women," *Journal of the American Medical Association*, 227 (1997): 1287–1292.

21. Lee and Paffenbarger.
22. Blair et al.
23. *Physical Activity and Health.*
24. Lee and Paffenbarger.
25. Blair et al.
26. AHA.
27. AHA.
28. AHA.
29. W. Haskill, "Physical Activity, Sport, and Health: Toward the Next Century," *Research Quarterly for Exercise and Sport,* 67 (Supplement to No. 3) (Sept. 1996), 537–547.
30. R. Klesges et al. "Effects of Television on Metabolic Rate: Potential Implications for Childhood Obesity," *Pediatrics,* 91 (1993): 281–286.
31. "Most Less Active Americans Want to be More Active," *NASPE News,* Winter, 1994, p. 11.
32. Klesges.
33. *CDC, Physical Activity and Health.*
34. Ibid.

Motivation and Motivational Techniques

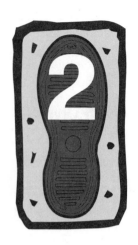

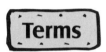

Terms

External (extrinsic) rewards
Internal (intrinsic) rewards
Positive feedback
Reinforcement
Self-motivation
Transtheoretical model for
    behavior change

Motivating people to begin and maintain an active way of life is a formidable and perplexing task. Although much has been said and written about the value of exercise, only 22% of people living in the United States are active enough to improve their health status.[1] After three decades into the exercise movement, the majority of Americans are essentially sedentary. Some are not convinced of the value of exercise. Others are unaware of its value. Still others would rather be sedentary regardless.

MOVING TOWARD AN ACTIVE LIFESTYLE

Motivating people to begin exercising is indeed difficult, and keeping them exercising after they begin is even more difficult. The exercise dropout rate is 50% during the initial 6 months,[2] most of whom discontinue their exercise programs during the first 3 months,[3] and 70% to 80% drop out before the end of the first year.[4] Changing behavior is a complex phenomenon. Though many theories and models seek to explain and describe the process, scientists still are unable to predict with a high degree of accuracy who will succeed. No single theory or model will work for everyone because each individual is unique, with unique circumstances and needs. The models are not all-encompassing, and all of the factors involved in behavior change have yet to be identified.

COMPONENTS OF BEHAVIOR CHANGE

Research has suggested that exercise and physical activities consist of behaviors that are more complex than other health-related behaviors. Although exercise has some dimensions in common with other health behaviors, it is inherently unique, separating it from the other behaviors. Researchers continue to attempt to develop a model of behavior applicable to exercise that will enable them to identify potential dropouts and individuals who will persevere. If potential dropouts can be identified early, they can be targeted for appropriate intervention that might increase the probability of adherence.

One of the personality traits associated with adherence is **self-motivation**, the desire to persist at a task without constant help or praise. Exercisers in this category tend to (a) set short-term goals that are attainable, (b) select activities they enjoy, (c) keep the workout manageable in terms of time and effort required, and (d) join a group for a portion or the entirety of a workout.[5]

The reasons that exercise dropouts offer most often are lack of time, inconvenient or inaccessible exercise site, work conflicts, and poor spousal support.[6] They also cite situational factors, such as the travel requirements of their jobs, as impediments to regular participation.

Determining whether these barriers to exercise are actual or perceived is difficult. Exercise adherers often live farther away from the exercise facility and have no more leisure time than dropouts do. Support from mates repeatedly has been shown to be a predictor of exercise adherence, but some adherers indicate that it is less important than other factors. Perhaps one of the differences between those who continue to exercise and those who don't is that the dropouts perceive impediments to exercise as real barriers.

Adherers perceive these same barriers as mere inconveniences that they can easily surmount. Turning dropouts into adherers, therefore, might be accomplished by changing dropouts' perceptions. Providing instruction in time management and flexible exercise hours and developing home exercise programs for these people might be productive.

Some generalizations regarding exercise adherence are as follows:[7]

1. Blue-collar workers, smokers, and obese people are less likely to begin and sustain exercise in either a supervised or an individual program.

2. People who are highly self-motivated are more likely to continue unsupervised exercise.

3. Perceptions of lack of time and inconvenience lead to dropping out, but some exercisers continue despite the same barriers.

4. Reinforcement from health and exercise professionals, support from significant others, feelings of well-being, and attainment of goals seem to be important factors in continuation of exercise.

Learning theories indicate that the assimilation of new and complicated patterns of behaviors, such as moving from a sedentary lifestyle to a more active one, might require an incremental approach to attain the desired behavior.[8] For example, if the long-range goal is to walk 45 minutes a day, the person might begin with 15-minute daily walks. When the exerciser adjusts and becomes comfortable with this level of energy expenditure, 5 minutes could be added each week to the daily walk until achieving the target. At this point, the exerciser might be satisfied to continue this level of exercise for a lifetime (maintenance) or he or she might establish a different, more difficult goal. The success associated with accomplishing the first goal will contribute to attaining the second.

Adhering to the program depends substantially on the reinforcement or rewards they receive from participation in exercise. Rewards can take many forms. A reward can be **extrinsic** (external) **reinforcement** or **intrinsic** (internal) **reinforcement,** or it might have physical parameters. Receiving praise and encouragement from others for example, are extrinsic rewards. A feeling of accomplishment for reaching a goal that required commitment and effort is an intrinsic reward. A gain in muscle, loss of fat, and an increase in energy are examples of the physical benefits that result from exercise. Any or all of these forms of **positive feedback** can provide the incentive and motivation for persisting in the program.[9] The new exercise behavior, which requires time and effort to sustain, will have to compete with or replace former sedentary behaviors that also were satisfying and rewarding, such as watching television and "surfing the net."

The ultimate goal is to participate consistently in deliberately conceived physical activities such as jogging, cycling, rowing, cross-country skiing, swimming, weight training, and the like. On the way to achieving this goal, we should take advantage of the opportunities in our daily lives to increase the level and frequency of our energy expenditure by doing chores such as mowing the lawn, washing and waxing the car by hand, taking the stairs instead of escalators and elevators, walking instead of driving, and many others. Lifestyle changes such as these do not happen overnight.

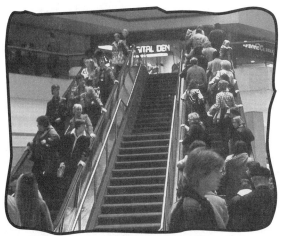

People would benefit from taking stairs instead of escalators.

It is disappointing that the public has not responded much to the Surgeon General's report on the importance of physical activity for improving health, preventing disease, and increasing longevity. The electronic media — television in particular — has been used successfully on occasion to change health behavior. Two decades ago the tobacco companies were advertising their products heavily through this medium and sales were robust and increasing. The ads were glitzy, glamorous, sexy, and targeted to teenagers and young adults. In response to pressure from health professionals and other concerned citizens regarding the lack of a rebuttal to the proliferation of smoking ads on television, Congress enacted a fairness doctrine or equal-time law compelling the television industry to provide time for anti-smoking commercials. It took only 2 years for these commercials to erode cigarette sales significantly. The result was that the tobacco companies voluntarily and wisely removed all tobacco ads from TV.

This move accomplished two important things for the tobacco industry: (a) Cigarette sales increased the year after the ads were removed, and (b) the equal-time concept was nullified so the anti-smoking commercials dried up as well. The tobacco companies transferred their advertising dollars to various forms of the print media and sponsorship of sporting events, while the anti-smoking messages had no place to go.

The point is that people who watch television sometimes act upon what they are exposed to. The anti-smoking messages worked. Further, in July 1996, the Surgeon General's report was released amid a great deal of fanfare. TV newscasters introduced the report nationally and locally. It was discussed on TV news magazine shows and on morning news and entertainment shows. This report extolled the virtues of *moderate* physical activity. Vigorous exercise is not necessary to improve health. Activities that are a part of daily living can enhance health if these are done at an intensity level equal to walking 3 to 4 miles per hour. This message should have resonated with the public. Instead, it generated about as much interest and excitement as announcing that "the sky is blue."

One year after the Surgeon General's report was issued, the National Coalition for Promoting Physical Activity commissioned a national survey regarding the public's knowledge of physical activity and its benefits.[10] Some of the highlights are:

1. Only one-third of those surveyed were aware of the Surgeon General's report.

2. More than half were unaware that exercise has a cumulative effect, that it can be dispersed throughout the day and still produce health benefits.

3. At least 25% stated that they would *like* to be more active.

4. More than one-third are marginally active, a level that is not active enough to improve health.

A nationally sponsored survey commissioned by the editors of *Parade Magazine* found that half of Americans do not exercise, but 87% of them said they should.[11] Commenting on the U.S. lifestyle, Nancy Dickey, M.D., President Elect of the American Medical Association, said, "In terms of awareness and knowing about good health, I'd give Americans an A-minus or B-plus. But in terms of doing what we know we should, most of us —myself included — deserve only a C or a C-minus."

If we could distill into pill form the physiological, health, psychological, and emotional benefits derived from exercise, Americans would line up and pay any reasonable amount of money to get it. Yet, all of these benefits are there for the taking if we are willing to devote the time and effort to get them.

In an effort to inform and motivate Americans to become active, the Centers for Disease Control and Prevention (CDC) has developed a program entitled, "Physical Activity: It's Everywhere You Go." The program and its materials (three manuals, television messages from Olympic speed skater Dan Jansen, ads, and posters) are designed for health professionals and community leaders so they can effectively spread the word at the grassroots level.

The National Association for Sport and Physical Education (NASPE) has developed 30-second and 60-second public service announcements for television, to educate the public about the importance of developing and delivering quality physical education programs in the public schools.[12] Former Surgeon General C. Everett Koop showed his support for this effort by signing the cover letter that was sent to 210 TV stations throughout the United States. Time will tell whether these initiatives and others like them will be successful.

The electronic media have the potential to reach large numbers of people quickly. Even if the message is received, it might not be acted upon, even when that message comes from several of the most prestigious and influential health agencies in the country. Unfortunately, though attaining knowledge is a necessary first step, it does not necessarily result in action.

In one interesting theory, the transtheoretical model, behavior change is seen as a five-stage process.[13] (Figure 2.1).

1. *Precontemplation.* Applied to exercise, individuals at this first stage are not exercising. They probably are not considering exercising, and they might be denying that exercise should be part of their lifestyle. People in this stage need a solid reason to change their behavior. One approach would be to encourage them to move slowly along the continuum of stages instead of attempting to thrust themselves directly into the action stage.[14] Understanding why physical activity is important, that it promotes health enhancement and an improved quality of life, leads to the next stage.

2. *Contemplation.* Knowledge, or some other motivator such as, "It's time to lose a few pounds" or "My 48-year-old neighbor died of a heart attack this morning and I'm his age," could be stimulus enough for an individual to seriously consider starting an

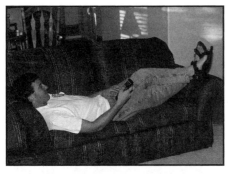

Stage 1: Precontemplation

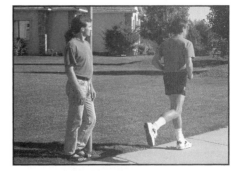

Stage 2: Contemplation

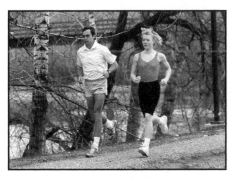

Stage 4: Action

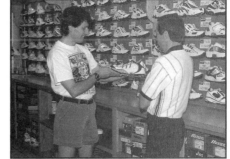

Stage 3: Preparation

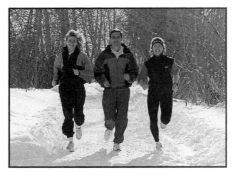

Stage 5: Maintenance

Figure 2.1 Stages in transtheoritical model.

exercise program. When this happens, the individual has progressed to the contemplation stage.

3. *Preparation.* At this stage the person demonstrates some overt movement signaling an intent to exercise, such as purchasing fitness equipment or a pair of walking/running shoes or joining a health club.

4. *Action.* The person finally arrives at this stage when he or she actually becomes involved in some physical activity. If this behavior change is successful, the person adheres to the program for some time.

5. *Maintenance.* Maintaining an exercise regimen does not guarantee that the exercise program will continue for life. People backslide for various reasons, and some drop out even after they have participated for a long time.

The time a person spends in any stage varies, and he or she might move back and forth among the stages. This model is a workable approach to changing behavior, but it does not work for all people, nor does it assure that a person will sustain the new behavior. People who drop out or backslide, however, can take comfort in the fact that the more attempts they make to establish a behavior change — in this case, lifetime exercise — the greater is the probability of eventual success.

Some psychologists have determined that a moderate level of motivation is optimal. Too little is likely to result in early failure, and too much may result in injury and burnout. In either case, motivation is affected adversely, adherence wanes, and the program, with all its good intentions and potential benefits, is terminated. This is graphically depicted by the inverted U hypothesis in Figure 2.2.

To avert this all-too-familiar scenario, we should approach our health and fitness goals slowly and patiently, albeit progressively. We must learn to contain our enthusiasm so as not to attempt too much too soon during the early phases of the program. Physical fitness is not

> Even the best laid plans sometimes go awry, and forces beyond your control interfere with the exercise program. Injuries and illnesses, job responsibilities, job-related travel, family and other obligations could interrupt your exercise program. If exercise is truly a priority in your life, though, you can surmount these barriers and find the time and the means to resume exercise.

achieved after only 2 weeks of training. Developing and maintaining physical fitness is a lifelong endeavor. It requires a sizable commitment of time and effort, but the results are eminently worthwhile. You supply the time and effort, and this text will provide you with the necessary knowledge. Appropriate application of these ingredients will increase your likelihood of success.

Factors that are motivating to one person may not have the same effect upon another because of differences in experience, interests, aims, objectives, intelligence, and many other factors. Therefore, selecting the precise factor or factors that will motivate any given individual to participate in a long-term walking or jogging program is conjectural at best.

Most people become involved with exercise for health-related reasons such as weight loss, reduction of stress and anxiety, prevention or delay of heart disease, muscle strength, a desire to live better and longer, or to sleep more restfully. The original reason for participation often becomes the primary reinforcer for maintaining the program. In some instances, the original reason is blended with others or assumes lesser importance as the person progresses and new goals assume greater priority.

Being knowledgeable about the beneficial health effects of exercise usually is not enough

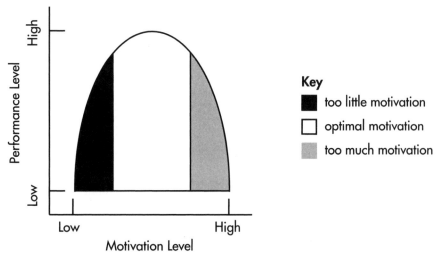

Figure 2.2 Inverted U hypothesis.

of a motivator for many people. Most people know that exercise is good for health, yet the majority don't participate. Knowledge is simply not enough to stimulate people to make positive behavioral changes. For instance, millions of people know that smoking cigarettes is harmful to their health, yet they continue to smoke.

We have at our disposal a variety of techniques that may motivate us to continue exercising. These help, in a general way, to maintain enthusiasm for a physically active life. Predicting the precise motive that will stimulate a specific individual to exercise, however, remains elusive.

SOME MOTIVATIONAL STRATEGIES

The following are practical suggestions to help people begin and continue an exercise program. Not every suggestion will appeal to every person. Still, one or more of these ideas might stimulate a person toward a lifestyle that includes exercise.

Develop a Knowledge Base

Understanding the need for exercise, as well as the associated health-related benefits, is a sufficient stimulus for some people to act, but it

is inadequate for most sedentary individuals. Nonetheless, Ken Cooper's first book motivated millions of sedentary Americans to become physically active.[15] Knowledge provides a rationale for an active life, and for those who respond positively to cognitive information, it might be a key motivator. As such, it is a technique commonly employed to enhance adherence to exercise.

Set Realistic Goals

Set goals for exercise that are specific and attainable. These should address the major accomplishments you will attempt to achieve. Goals might be weight control, muscle development, an increase in energy reserves, management of stress, reductions in serum cholesterol or blood pressure, prevention of chronic disease, or competition in road races. Walking and jogging, or a combination of the two, are effective exercise modalities for achieving all of these goals.

Novices might walk for 20 to 30 minutes per day, 4 to 5 days per week. Beginning joggers should jog for about 20 minutes per day three times per week. This does not include the time required for warming up and cooling down. Beginning joggers should ease into jogging by combining it with walking to diminish the musculoskeletal and cardiorespiratory stress. As fitness improves, walking time should be reduced while jogging time increases progressively to fill the entire 20 minutes. Speed should not be increased during this time. Jogging every other day will result in enough rest between exercise sessions for the body to fully recover.

As fitness improves, walkers can exercise more often (frequency) and for a longer time (duration). Because walking is a low-impact activity, it imposes less demand upon the musculoskeletal system than does jogging. The intensity of walking, however, should reflect a pace that is well tolerated and enables recovery from one workout to the next. Reasonable exercise and health goals should be selected within these parameters. Exercisers should be patient and not attempt or expect too much too soon. Exercising beyond one's capacity will produce discomfort and pain and could produce an injury. Any or all of these occurrences is likely to lead to discouragement, and ultimately to dropping out.

Select the Social Contexts That Are Most Supportive

People can choose where and with whom they will exercise. Whether to exercise alone or with others depends upon one's preference, personality, exercise needs and goals, and compatibility with other exercisers. Evidence is available to support both approaches, and each has advantages.

Attractive features of the group approach include camaraderie, the possibility of developing productive social relationships with other group members, cooperation, competition, and reinforcement. The social support received from the group, particularly during the early weeks of a beginner's program, enhances compliance.[16] Other people find that the individual approach to exercise is best for them. A 1-year study of older men and women showed that an individual home-based exercise program was more effective than a group program in promoting their adherence to exercise.[17] The researchers

found that the group exercise program was too inconvenient over the course of the year. Convenience and accessibility of the exercise facility were important considerations that affected adherence to the group program. Unless these two factors are resolved satisfactorily, the independent approach might be best for that population as a whole.

Exercise with a Buddy

Two people with similar training routines and compatible levels of physical fitness can provide motivational support for each other. Buddies can exchange knowledge about fitness training, nutrition, and a host of other topics of common interest to them. A bonus of the buddy system is that it becomes more difficult to skip a workout, even when the person would rather do something else, when someone is waiting at a designated time and place.

Enlist the Support of Those Who Are Important to You

Friends, mates, other family members, and co-workers — people with whom you interact frequently and whose advice you value — can be important sources of motivation, encouragement, and reinforcement. These people provide support by projecting a favorable attitude toward your exercising. A number of studies have shown that spousal support is particularly influential.

The support others provide is more effective when they themselves are exercisers. As such, they function as role models who can draw upon their knowledge and experiences to assist and provide advice. Occasionally working out with the new exerciser also helps.

Associate with Other Exercisers

Associating with other exercisers allows a person to catch their enthusiasm and also give them some. When people who exercise get together, their enthusiasm is highly visible. Walkers and joggers are eager to talk about their knowledge and experiences. Participants will gain new ideas and techniques that will motivate toward continuation of exercise.

Build on Successful Experiences

The importance of consistent exercise rather than superior performance should be emphasized. Developing physical fitness and enhancing health take time and patience. Some beneficial changes should begin to appear within the first 3 to 4 weeks. These can become a springboard for further gains.

Keep a Progress Chart

Keeping a daily record is helpful because this written information objectively shows the rate and amount of progress achieved. Looking back at the record and observing the gains can be a source of motivation when a person becomes discouraged. The chart should reflect body weight, type, amount, and duration of exercise, as well as resting and exercise heart rates. (See Chapter 4 for complete discussion.) The chart should allow room for comments. Figure 2.3 provides a form for keeping track of progress.

Weighing oneself before and after the workout is important, particularly in hot weather when fluid loss can become a major problem.

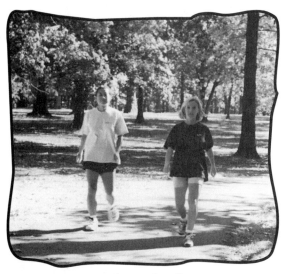

Normal gaited walking.

Most of the weight lost during the workout is liquid, so the difference between pre- and post-exercise weight is an approximation of the amount of fluid loss. A body weight loss of 2% is indicative of slight dehydration.[18] A 3% loss is still safe, a 5% loss is considered borderline, and an 8% loss is dangerous.[19] The loss of 1 pound of body weight is approximately equal to 1 pint of fluid loss.

Determining or approximating fluid loss is one of the functional aspects of the progress chart. Over the long term, trends in weight loss, distance covered, and heart rates (exercise and resting) will become discernible, and a record of improvement will become apparent.

Exercise to Music

Music can provide the motivation to continue exercising, as well as providing rhythm, and it tends to take the mind off the effort associated with walking and jogging.[20] A researcher at Ohio State University tested experienced runners with and without upbeat music.[21] The runners stated that music made the exercise bout seem easier. The researchers ran both trials, one with and one without music, at the same workload. Measures of working heart rate and blood lactate indicated that the runners were working equally hard on both trials; only their perceptions of the difficulty of the workload had changed. Music can be provided easily indoors, and portable radio headsets are popular among outdoor walkers and joggers.

Set a Definite Time and Place for Exercise

The exerciser should set a definite time and a convenient place during the early stages of the exercise program, resolving to walk or jog at least three times per week. The exerciser should schedule the workout just as any other important activity. Temptations should be resisted to replace the workout with some other pursuit that is more appealing. Skipping workouts becomes habit-forming quickly; the more you do it, the easier it becomes. After becoming hooked

DATE	BODY WEIGHT		EXERCISE			INTENSITY**			COMMENTS
	Pre-Exercise	Post-Exercise	Type	Duration*		RHR	THR	PE	

*Time, distance, etc.
**RHR = resting heart rate; THR = training heart rate; PE = perceived exertion

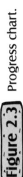 **Figure 2.3** Progress chart.

on exercise (it takes 3 to 6 months), the time and place can be varied to meet changing environmental conditions (weather that is too hot, too humid, too wet, too cold, and so on), work schedules, and other conflicting responsibilities.

When is the best time of day to work out? The best time seems to be immediately at the end of the workday and before dinner. This serves two purposes:

1. It metabolizes the stress products that have accumulated in the blood during the day.
2. It temporarily suppresses the appetite, resulting in the consumption of fewer calories at dinner.

If lack of time is resulting in missed workouts, the exerciser might try exercising less frequently but more intensely. Although this approach increases the potential for injury, it is better than abandoning the program completely. Exercising fewer than three times per week will not increase the fitness level but will lessen the impact of detraining. Upon returning to the normal exercise routine, the fitness level will not have deteriorated to the point of having to start from scratch.

Focus on the Positives

Novice exercisers rather quickly become aware of the negatives associated with working out — among them, muscle soreness, amount of effort required, sweating, and the feeling of fatigue. These factors should not act as deterrents. The exerciser should concentrate, instead, on accomplishments — the sense of relaxation after exercise, the increase in energy reserves, the loss of body fat and gain in muscle tissue, improvement in physical appearance, better health, improved self-concept, and overall feeling of well-being. Focusing on the positives will help keep a person motivated and excited about exercise.

Don't Become Obsessive About Exercise

Exercise should consist of activities that are fun and enjoyable and also allow you to reach your goals. Exercise should be relaxing and recreational but not obstructive. If a person feels and acts miserable after missing a day of exercise, this is obsessive. Sometimes unplanned circumstances don't allow a person to exercise on a given day. When that happens, it can be considered as one of the two days of rest included in the exercise agenda and picked up tomorrow or the next day. People should not exercise when they are ill. Missing an occasional workout will not detract from the fitness benefits already achieved. Activity can be resumed upon recovery. Later in this text you will learn about the importance of rest to an exercise program.

NO EXERCISE FAILURES

Physical fitness and health enhancement can be achieved and maintained without competing against others or the time clock. The exercise program that is ultimately adopted should be enjoyable and comfortable, and it should fit the exerciser's level of physical fitness. Walking and jogging are not complex skills. And in these noncompetitive venues, there are no last-place finishes to worry about, no embarrassment with performance, and no intimidation from others.

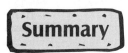

Summary

- Only 22% of Americans are active enough to improve their health status.
- The exercise dropout rate is 50% during the first 6 months after exercise begins.
- Most of the "least active" Americans don't exercise because of lack of time, work conflicts, travel requirements of the job, inconvenient or inaccessible exercise site, and poor support from family members, among other reasons.
- Blue-collar workers, smokers, and obese people are less likely than others to begin and sustain exercise.
- External rewards are effective in the early phase of the exercise program, and internal rewards are best for maintaining exercise.

◆ People can take advantage of opportunities in daily life to increase energy expenditure — by mowing the lawn, washing and waxing the car, taking the stairs instead of elevators and escalators, and so on.

◆ The Surgeon General's report on the importance of exercise for improving health has not motivated most sedentary people to exercise.

◆ Only moderate levels of exercise are needed to improve health; this can be accomplished by walking three or four times a week.

◆ The transtheoretical model of behavior has useful potential in motivating sedentary people to become active and maintain an exercise program.

◆ A moderate level of motivation is optimal — too little exercise is likely to result in failure, and too much can result in injury and burnout.

◆ Most people concede that exercise is good for enhancing health and improving physical appearance, but the majority of them don't participate.

◆ Goals for exercise should be realistic, specific, and attainable.

◆ Walking is a low-impact activity that imposes less demand than jogging on the musculoskeletal system.

◆ Though exercising with a group has a number of advantages, some people prefer to exercise on their own.

◆ Exercise buddies can motivate each other and exchange knowledge regarding physical fitness.

◆ Spouses, other family members, friends, and co-workers can be important sources of motivation, encouragement, and reinforcement.

◆ Emphasize the importance of exercising consistently rather than stressing superior exercise performance.

Notes

1. Centers for Disease Control and Prevention, *Physical Activity and Health: A Report of the Surgeon General* (Atlanta: National Center for Chronic Disease Prevention and Health Promotion, 1996).
2. A.C. King, and M. Kiernan, "Physical Activity Promotion: Antecedents," *ACSM's Resource Manual for Guidelines for Exercise Testing and Prescription*, 3d edition, edited by J. L. Roitman (Baltimore: Williams and Wilkins, 1998).
3. R. Dishman and J. Sallis, "Determinants and Interventions for Physical Activity and Exercise," in *Physical Activity, Fitness, and Health*, edited by C. Bouchard, et al. (Champaign, IL: Human Kinetics Publishers, 1994).
4. King and Kiernan.
5. J.J. Annesi, "Relevant Retention Research," *Fitness Management*, 12:10 (Sept. 1996), 42–43.
6. R.K. Dishman and J. Buckworth, "Increasing Physical Activity: A Quantitative Synthesis," *Medicine and Science in Sports and Exercise*, 28 (1996), 706–719.
7. Dishman and Sallis.
8. National Center for Chronic Disease Prevention and Health Promotion, *Physical Activity and Health*
9. Ibid.
10. "How to Get Americans Active," *AAHPERD Update* (Sept./Oct. 1997).
11. M. Clements and D. Hales, "How Healthy Are We?" *Parade Magazine* (Sept. 7, 1997), 4–7.
12. "How to Get Americans Active."
13. B.A. Brehm, "Helping Clients Change," *Fitness Management*, 13:1 (Jan. 1997), 24–26.
14. Clements and Hales.
15. K. H. Cooper, *Aerobics*, (New York, NY: Bantam Books Inc., 1968).
16. CDC, *Physical Activity and Health*.
17. King and Kiernan.
18. T.E. Bernard, "Environmental Considerations: Heat and Cold," *ACSMs Resource Guide for Guidelines for Exercise Testing and Prescription*, 3d edition, edited by J.L. Roitman (Baltimore: Williams and Wilkins, 1998).
19. E. T. Howley and B.D. Franks, *Health Fitness Instructor's Handbook* (Champaign, IL: Human Kinetics, 1997).
20. Ibid.
21. R.J. Trotter, "Maybe It's The Music" *Psychology Today*, 8:19 (May, 1984).

Guidelines for Walking and Jogging

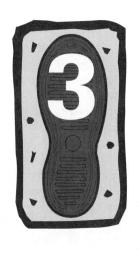

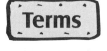

Terms

Aerobic capacity

Calisthenics

Cardiac reserve

Cardiorespiratory training effect

Cross-training

Duration

Dynamic/ballistic stretching

Exercise electrocardiogram (ECG)

Exercise heart rate

Frequency

Heart rate reserve

Intensity

Karvonen method

Kilocalories (kcals)

Maximal heart rate

Metabolic diseases

Myotatic reflex

Norepinephrine

Overload

Overtraining

Physical activity

Progression

Proprioceptive neuromuscular facilitation (PNF)

Rate of perceived exertion (RPE)

Resting heart rate

Specificity

Static stretching

Systolic blood pressure

Target heart rate

If walking and jogging are to have a significant and lasting impact on our state of health, they should become lifelong activities. A sound program, based upon the guidelines and suggestions presented in this text, has the capacity to improve both the quality and the quantity of one's life. The health benefits of walking and jogging will be discussed in Chapters 5 and 6. For now, we will focus on starting your program correctly, to increase the probability of success and thereby promote your adherence to exercise.

REGULAR AND CONSISTENT PARTICIPATION

To be effective, walking, jogging, or any other form of exercise must be performed regularly. Regular participation for 2 to 3 months will yield substantial physiological and psychological benefits that ultimately may provide the motivation to continue. The major challenge for the beginning exerciser is to sustain physical activity during the early weeks of participation without losing interest or becoming injured. Enthusiastic beginners, anxious to achieve their goals rapidly, tend to

27

overdo it in the early stage of their fitness program.

Beginners face a "catch-22" situation: They need enough motivation and enthusiasm to start and maintain the exercise habit, but too much enthusiasm can stimulate them to exercise beyond their capacity. Exercising beyond one's fitness level is not enjoyable. It is extremely uncomfortable and even potentially dangerous. If the exerciser attempts to push the program, negative feelings toward exercise will develop quickly, and soon the program, with all of its good intentions, will be discarded.

After all, how many of us are masochistic enough to endure discomfort and pain in every exercise session? Consistent participation comes about from our enjoyment of exercise. For typical people, pain and enjoyment are contradictory. Therefore, novices should not become overly impatient for rapid gains. These will come soon enough.

THE MEDICAL EXAM

Prior to beginning an exercise program, a medical examination is desirable for men 40 years of age and older, and for women 50 years of age and older.[1] People who are apparently healthy may participate in low- to moderate-intensity exercises without medical clearance. People who are at higher risk — those who have two or more major coronary risk factors or symptoms that suggest metabolic disease (for example, diabetes, kidney and liver disease) should have a medical exam that includes a physician-monitored **exercise electrocardiogram** (ECG). Young adults (college age) usually can start exercising without medical clearance. Everyone should begin within their capacity and progress gradually.

ACHIEVING OBJECTIVES

The exerciser's aims and objectives should help determine the direction of the program and the type of physical activity selected. Weight loss, road race competition, and the development of strength are objectives that suggest different types of physical activities as well as different exercise emphases. The objective of properly conceived exercise programs should be reflected by the manner in which the principles of exercise are utilized. The extent to which each is emphasized or deemphasized is the key to accomplishing specific objectives.

WARMING UP

Each exercise bout should be preceded by an 8- to 10-minute warm-up and followed by a cool-down period of equal time. Both are integral components of an exercise program. Proper warm-up and cool-down procedures contribute to performance and the exerciser's health and safety. Sandwiched between these two components is the actual exercise program — in this text, walking and jogging.

The warm-up is designed to prepare the body gradually for more vigorous exercise. In approximately 10 minutes of warming up, the muscles to be involved in the activity are heated, and the heart rate is allowed to increase slowly toward the rate expected during the actual workout. Rhythmic **calisthenics**, walking, slow jogging, and other low-intensity activities can be used during the warm-up to prepare the individual for exercise of greater intensity. These activities smooth the transition from inactivity to activity with minimum oxygen deprivation to the heart, muscles, and organs.

Without a proper warm-up, the heart rate would rise rapidly, forcing the body to rely upon short-term supplies of fuel to generate the energy needed for exercise. Circulation does not increase proportionately to heart rate, causing a brief interval of time (about 2 minutes) when the heart and other muscles are not fully supplied with oxygen. This is a potentially dangerous time, particularly for those whose circulation is compromised by heart and blood vessel disease.

An example of the healthy heart's response to exercise with and without warming up was illustrated in a study using 44 healthy male subjects ages 21 to 52.[2] All of the subjects had normal electrocardiographic (ECG) responses to running on a treadmill when they were allowed a warm-up of 2 minutes of easy jogging. When the same exercise was not preceded by a warm-up, 70% of the same group developed abnormal ECG responses.

When the cardiorespiratory warm-up phase is complete the muscles are stretched. At this point the walker or jogger should be sweating, indicating that the core temperature might be elevated slightly and muscle temperature is substantially elevated.[3] Both responses enhance performance and reduce the risk of physical injury. Muscles are stretched more effectively when they are heated.

Static stretching is the preferred method for enhancing and maintaining flexibility of the joints and elasticity of muscles and connective tissue. Static stretching consists of slow controlled movements and desired end positions that are held for 10 to 30 seconds.[4] The desired end position should produce a feeling of mild discomfort but not pain. If the stretch is painful, you are stretching too forcefully and are in danger of exceeding the elastic properties of muscles. Static stretching is effective because

— it is not likely to cause injury,
— it produces no muscle soreness,
— it helps to alleviate muscle soreness, and
— it requires little energy.

Static stretches are effective and convenient, they do not require the assistance of a partner, nor is any equipment necessary. Typical stretches for walking and jogging are illustrated in Figures 3.1 through 3.8.

Proprioceptive neuromuscular facilitation (PNF) has infiltrated the fitness movement as another technique for increasing flexibility. Physical therapists have used PNF stretching for many years for patients with neuromuscular disorders. PNF stretching is more effective than static stretching in improving flexibility,[5] but it has limitations.[6]

1. Most PNF techniques require the assistance of a partner who is competent in this system, so as not to injure the exerciser.

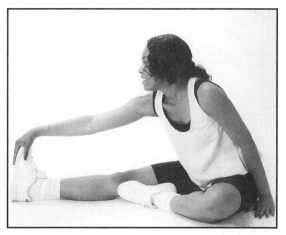

Figure 3.1 Modified Hurdler's Stretch. Sit with the right leg fully extended with the sole of the left foot against the inner right thigh. Keeping the right leg straight, lean forward as far as you can and attempt to reach your foot with the extended right arm. Hold 15 to 30 seconds and switch legs and arms. Stretches the hamstring muscle group in the backs of the thighs.

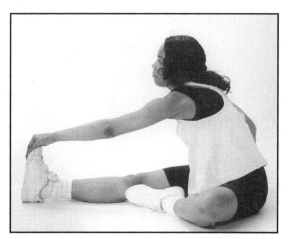

Figure 3.2 Modified Hurdler's Stretch. Similar to Figure 3.1 but slightly more challenging in that you reach forward with the opposite hand. This will place some stretch on the lower back. Hold 15 to 30 seconds, then switch legs and arms.

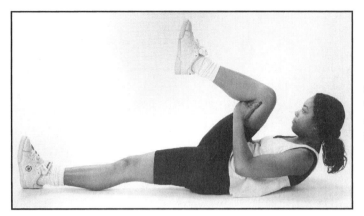

Figure 3.3 Back Stretcher. Lie on your back with hands clasped at the back of the thigh of your right leg. Pull your leg to your chest and hold for 15 to 30 seconds. Switch legs. Stretches the lower back.

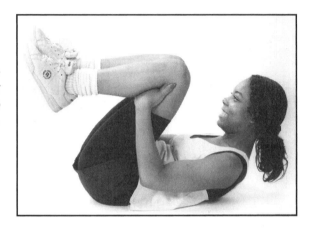

Figure 3.4 Back Stretcher. From the same position as Figure 3.3, clasp your hands behind both thighs and pull both legs to your chest and hold for 15 to 30 seconds. Stretches the lower back.

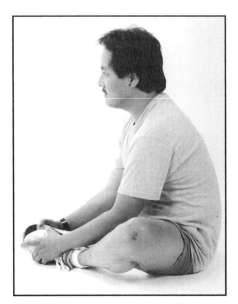

Figure 3.5 Stretching the Inner Thighs and Hips. Seated, bend your knees so the soles of the feet come together. Use your forearms to push your knees toward the floor. Hold 15 to 30 seconds.

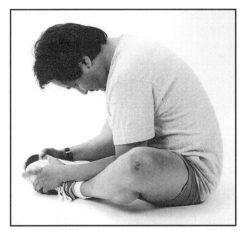

Figure 3.6 Stretching the Inner Thighs and Hips. A variation of the exercise in Figure 3.5. In this case, lean forward as you push the knees to the floor. Hold 15 to 30 seconds.

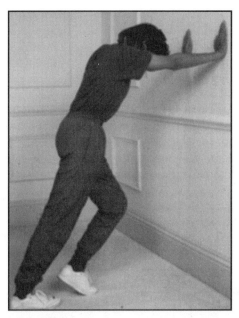

Figure 3.8 Achilles Tendon Stretch. Assume a stride position with the forward leg bent at the knee. The rear leg is straight with the heel planted firmly on the floor. Lean forward until you feel the stretch in the calf and achilles tendon above the heel. Hold 15 to 30 seconds. Switch legs. Be sure to point your feet straight ahead.

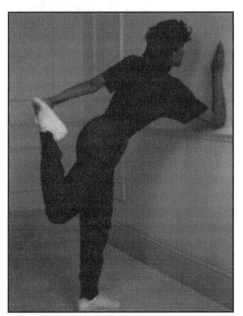

Figure 3.7 Thigh Stretcher. Bend your right leg and pull that foot upward with the opposite hand to avoid excessive bend at the knee. Hold 15 to 30 seconds. Switch legs and hands. You may use the opposite hand to maintain balance. Stretches the quadriceps muscle group at the front of the thighs.

2. Using PNF techniques takes more time.
3. PNF is associated with more pain and muscle stiffness.
4. PNF techniques are more complex than static stretching procedures.

For these reasons, even though PNF stretching is slightly more effective than static stretching, it is not the preferable method.

Dynamic or **ballistic stretching** is not recommended because it forces muscles to pull against themselves. This type of stretching entails bouncing and bobbing movements that activate the **myotatic reflex**. Each rapid stretch sends a volley of signals from the stretch reflex to the central nervous system, which responds by ordering the stretching muscles to contract instead.

If you have dozed off while sitting in a chair, you probably have experienced the results of the stretch reflex responding to rapid stretch. Your head drops forward as you nod off, causing the neck muscles to stretch rapidly. This sudden dynamic stretch sets in motion the reflexive process that results in rapid contraction of the neck muscles and a quick return of the head to the upright position. The rapid movements in opposite directions can result in muscle soreness and possible injury.

PRINCIPLES OF EXERCISE

The six principles of exercise are intensity, frequency, duration, overload, progression, and specificity. These are discussed in turn.

Intensity

Intensity refers to the amount of energy expended per bout of exercise. For the development of physical fitness, the American College of Sports Medicine (ACSM) recommends an exercise intensity of 55/65% to 90% of maximum heart rate or 40/50% to 85% of the **cardiac reserve**.[7] Adults typically exercise at the low end of the range, whereas heart patients and healthy people with low functional capacity tend to exercise below the suggested range.[8]

The ACSM guidelines for health enhancement were issued in conjunction with the Centers For Disease Control and Prevention. According to these guidelines, a person does not have to exercise vigorously to improve health. **Physical activity** done at a moderate level is all that is necessary. Moderately intense physical activity consists of any activity that equals the amount of calories (energy) used to walk 3 to 4 miles per hour (mph).[9] This is a 15 to 20 minute-mile pace. When performed regularly, this activity can improve *health* by promoting weight loss and by lowering blood pressure and cholesterol levels. Exercise at this intensity, however, produces only minimum improvement in *physical fitness*.

Although health can improve through moderate, regular exercise, physical activities at higher intensities produce significant improvements in *both* physical fitness and health status.

Several methods can be used to determine the proper intensity for exercise. One of the most practical is the "talk test." If you cannot carry on a conversation fairly comfortably while walking or jogging, you might be exercising at a pace that is too intense for your level of fitness.

A second method involves your *perception* of the effort, called **rate of perceived exertion (RPE)**. Perceived exertion is an excellent method for monitoring exercise because it includes significant indicators of effort other than heart rate. For example it includes overall exertional discomfort and fatigue, rate and depth of breathing, muscle fatigue, and body temperature. These are your subjective impressions of the effort that encompasses sensory input from all of the systems associated with generation of energy for movement. The Borg Rate of Perceived Exertion Scale (RPE) and the revised Category-Ratio RPE Scale appear in Figure 3.9.

These scales provide exercisers of all fitness levels with guidelines for selecting the appropriate intensity based on their subjective perceptions of their effort. The **cardiorespiratory training effect** begins at an RPE of 12 to 13 (somewhat hard) on the original scale and 4 (somewhat strong) on the newer scale. Exercise intensities above these values will lead to the production and accumulation of lactic acid and exercise discomfort. Lactic acid is a fatiguing metabolite resulting from the incomplete breakdown of glucose (sugar). Build-up of lactic acid in the exercising muscles produces fatigue and interferes with the muscle's ability to contract and continue to perform physical work at the same level.[10]

Values of 12 to 14 on the original RPE scale and 4 on the new scale, approximate 60% to 80% of the **aerobic capacity**, 60% to 80% of the **heart rate reserve** (also known as cardiac reserve), and 70% to 85% of the **maximal heart rate**. The latter two concepts are explained in the following section.

A third method for monitoring exercise is by **exercise heart rate** or **target heart rate (HR)**. Exercise heart rate can be determined in two ways. The first uses a percentage of the maximum heart rate, and the second uses a percentage of the heart rate reserve. The estimated maximum heart rate (HR max) must be determined as a first step for each method. This is accomplished by subtracting your age in years from the constant 220. Thus, the HR max for a 20-year-old would be:

$$\begin{array}{rl} 220 & \text{(Constant)} \\ -20 & \text{(Age)} \\ \hline 200 & \text{bpm (HR max)} \end{array}$$

The HR max decreases with age, so the value for a 50-year-old would be 170 bpm ($220 - 50 = 170$ bpm). Regardless of age, this method is only an estimate of the HR max. The HR that the exerciser will attempt to maintain during exercise is referred to as the target HR.

The first method for establishing the target HR uses a percentage of the HR max. The ACSM recommends that people exercise at an intensity level somewhere between 55/65% and 90% of HR max. A person in average physical condition would select the middle of the range, or 70% to 80% of the HR max. Our 20-year-old with a HR max of 200 bpm would have a target HR of 140 bpm to 160 bpm. This is computed as follows:

$$\begin{array}{rl} 200 \text{ bpm (HR max)} \\ \times .7 \\ \hline 140 \text{ bpm} \end{array} \qquad \begin{array}{rl} 200 \text{ bpm (HR max)} \\ \times .8 \\ \hline 160 \text{ bpm} \end{array}$$

People who are in better physical condition would select a higher percentage of their HR max, and those in poorer condition would select a lower percentage.

A more sophisticated approach for determining target HR is by the **Karvonen method**. This method employs the exerciser's **resting heart rate**, which is a crude measure of physical fitness, and the cardiac reserve, which is the difference between the HR max and the resting HR. Fit people in general have lower resting

Category RPE Scale		Category-Ratio RPE Scale	
6		0	Nothing at all
7	Very, very light	0.5	Very, very weak
8		1	Very weak
9	Very light	2	Weak
10		3	Moderate
11	Fairly light	4	Somewhat strong
12		5	Strong
13	Somewhat hard	6	
14		7	Very strong
15	Hard	8	
16		9	
17	Very hard	10	Very, very strong
18		•	Maximal
19	Very, very hard		
20			

From G. A. V. Borg, *Medicine and Science in Sports and Exercise, 14* (1982), 377–387.

Figure 3.9 Borg's RPE scales — original scale on the left; revised scale on the right.

HRs and higher cardiac reserves than unfit people. The target for a 20-year-old in average physical condition with a resting HR of 70 bpm is calculated in the following manner using the Karvonen method:

1. Calculate HR max as before:

$$\begin{array}{r} 220 \\ -20 \\ \hline 200 \end{array} \text{ bpm (HR max)}$$

2. The Karvonen formula is:

THR = cardiac reserve × TI% + RHR
Where:
THR = target heart rate
Cardiac reserve = HR max − RHR
TI% = training intensity
(Get this value from Table 3.1.)
RHR = resting heart rate
Therefore:
THR = (HR max − RHR) × TI% + RHR
= (200 − 70) × .70 + 70
= 161 bpm

To use the Karvonen method, the resting HR must be known. According to the American College of Sports Medicine, the resting heart rate should be taken in the standing position.

Learning to take HR by palpating the pulse is a skill that must be developed. The two most practical sites — and the ones most often used — are at the radial and carotid arteries, illustrated in Figures 3.10 and 3.11. The radial pulse is palpated at the thumb side of the wrist with the hand held palm up. The carotid pulse is felt in the large artery at either side of the neck. The

first two fingers of either hand are used to count the pulse rate in either location.

Because the arteries in the neck are sensitive to pressure, care should be taken when palpating the carotid pulse. Excessive pressure stretches the arteries and stimulates specialized receptors therein that respond reflexively by slowing the heart's rate of beating. This leads to

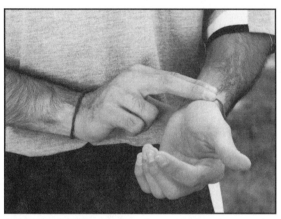

Figure 3.10 Taking the radial pulse at the wrist with the fingers.

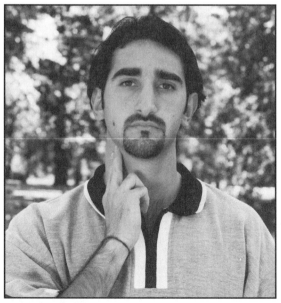

Figure 3.11 Taking the carotid pulse at the neck.

Table 3.1 Guidelines for Selecting Training Intensity Level

Fitness Level	Intensity Level (%)
Low	60
Fair	65
Average	70
Good	75
Excellent	80–90

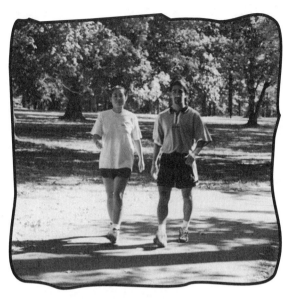

Strolling is casual walking at a pace of 3 miles per hour or slower.

underestimation of the actual heart rate. To circumvent this effect, the pressure applied to the carotid should not exceed the amount required to feel the pulse. To estimate the heart rate in beats per minute, count the number of pulse beats for 15 seconds and multiply that number by 4.

Frequency

Frequency refers to the number of times per week that a person participates in physical activity. The development of physical fitness requires that the individual exercise 3 to 5 days per week at the appropriate level of intensity.[11] Fewer than 3 days per week is not enough of a stimulus to improve fitness, and more than 5 days per week results in diminishing returns, staleness, and increases the likelihood of injury. If health improvement is the goal, however, low-intensity exercise of moderate duration (20 to 40 minutes), such as strolling (walking at 3 mph) could be done every day without resulting in orthopedic problems or staleness.

A person does not have to exercise in one continuous bout to gain benefits from it. Exercise can be split into several shorter sessions during the day. Two groups of male subjects exercised for a total of 30 minutes a day, three times per week, at 65% to 75% of their HR max.[12] One of the groups exercised continuously for 30 minutes, and the other group split the 30 minutes into three 10-minute exercise sessions. At the end of 8 weeks, the fitness level of both groups improved, but the one-exercise session group improved more. During the course of the study, however, both groups lost the same amount of weight. Short bouts of exercise spaced throughout the day is a realistic exercise option for busy people.

Days of rest are an important component of any training program. They are needed for physical and mental recuperation. Exercisers who don't take days off run the risk of burning out or becoming stale. There is a fine line between the amount of exercise that produces maximum gains and the amount of exercise that results in the negative effects (staleness) associated with **overtraining**. Signs of overtraining are:

1. A feeling of chronic fatigue and listlessness
2. Inability to make further fitness gains (or even a loss of fitness)
3. Sudden loss of weight
4. An increase of 5 beats or more in the resting heart rate, taken in the morning prior to getting out of bed
5. Loss of enthusiasm for working out (the exerciser no longer looks forward to the workout)
6. Vulnerability to injury and illness
7. Generalized anger
8. Depression.

Staleness can be both psychological (lack of variety in the program or boredom after years of training) and physiological. Regardless, the treatment is the same: Either stop training for a few days to a few weeks (depending upon the severity of staleness) or cut back substantially. In either case, rebuild and regain fitness gradually. Prevention is the best treatment. Recognize the signs and adjust accordingly before staleness becomes a problem.

Duration

How long a person exercises is referred to as **duration**. In its latest guidelines, the ACSM recommended that exercise of low intensity should last a minimum of 30 minutes and be performed most days of the week.[13] This amount of exercise will improve the health status of all people and the fitness level of sedentary people. This should be considered a minimum program, though. Epidemiological data have shown that expending 1000 **kilocalories (kcals)** to 2000 kcals per week — the equivalent of walking or jogging 10 to 20 miles per week — resulted in fewer heart attacks and longer life.[14] To improve physical fitness measurably, the duration of exercise should be 20 to 60 minutes with the exercise heart rate in the appropriate zone (as determined by the Karvonen method), and the exerciser should participate 3 to 5 days per week.

Overload and Progression

Overload involves subjecting the various systems of the body (muscular, cardiorespiratory, skeletal) to greater physical demand. **Progression** is the manner and the time when these demands are applied. Periodically applying overload forces the body to adapt, and in the process, physical fitness is developed. To improve, exercisers must overload on a schedule of systematic progression. After attaining the desired level of fitness, the exerciser switches from the development of fitness to the maintenance of fitness. At this point, the practices of overload and progression no longer come into play.

Like other forms of exercise, overload can be applied systematically and progressively to walking and jogging. This can be accomplished by one or a combination of the following:

1. Gradually increase the distance.

2. Decrease the time that it takes to cover a specified distance.

3. Participate more frequently.

A good rule of thumb is to increase the frequency and duration of exercise while holding the intensity steady. After a base of fitness has been developed, intensity can be increased.

Three observations might be noted regarding the application of overload:

♦ Patience is necessary so as not to exercise beyond your capacity.

♦ Fitness improves the most during the first 3 months of training and continues for some time, but in smaller increments.

♦ Overload should be applied only when individuals are ready to accept a new challenge.

Specificity

The body adapts according to the specific type of stress to which it is subjected. This is referred to as **specificity**. The muscles, systems, and organs used in any activity adapt in the specific way in which they are used. Jogging does not prepare a person for swimming, nor does swimming prepare a person for cycling, because these activities are sufficiently different from each other. Jogging stresses the legs in a manner unique to that activity. The adaptations that result from jogging provide little carryover to the leg kick for swimming.

Competitors who are attempting to maximize their physical performance in a given activity are locked into a training program that is task-specific. This involves repetitive overloading of the muscles used in the event. Triathalon training provides a good example of the principle of specificity. Triathletes must train vigorously in all three events of the triathalon because no combination of training for any two of them will result in substantial improvement in the third.

People who walk or jog for health and fitness are not confined solely to these activities. They occasionally can swim, cycle, play tennis, racquetball, or other games for fun and variety. Although walking and jogging are the core of the fitness program, participants have the option of engaging in other activities on occasion if they desire.

At least 2 days of weight training are a must. Weight training should supplement walking and jogging because it stresses the total muscular system in ways that walking and jogging cannot achieve. Many people who exercise for health reasons enjoy participating in more than one physical activity. This is called **cross-training**. Still others prefer one activity because they enjoy it and it meets their needs. The point is to select an activity or activities that provide enjoyment and fulfill your health and fitness needs. Walking and jogging qualify for both.

COOLING DOWN AFTER EXERCISE

Cooling down after exercise is just as important as warming up. The body was allowed to speed up gradually, and it also must be allowed to slow down gradually. The body is not analogous to an auto engine that can be turned on and off with the twist of a key. Cool-down should last about 8 to 10 minutes. The first phase should consist of walking or some other light activity, and the second phase should consist of the same stretching exercises that were done during the warm-up.

Phase One: Light Activity

Five minutes of continuous light activity causes rhythmical muscle contractions that prevent the pooling of blood and help to move blood back to the heart for redistribution to the vital organs. This boost to circulation after exercise is essential to the cool-down. Inactivity during this time forces the heart to compensate for the reduced volume of blood returning to it by maintaining a high pumping rate. The recovery period following exercise represents a potential hazard if it is not approached properly. The

exerciser runs the risk of dizziness, fainting, and perhaps more serious consequences associated with diminished blood flow, the most serious of which is sudden death. Although sudden death during or immediately after exercise is rare, it does occur, and the recovery period is a likely time.

The worst possible cool-down procedure after fast walking or jogging is to stop all activity and stand still. The blood vessels in the legs that were dilated during exercise remain that way for a time after exercise, so blood pools in the leg veins. The downward force of gravity impedes the return of blood from the legs to the heart. Dilation of the blood vessels plus the force of gravity reduces blood flow to the heart, which limits the amount available for the body's various systems.

Because venous return of blood to the heart is reduced, the **systolic blood pressure** drops but heart rate remains high. The systolic pressure represents the pressure of the blood against the artery walls when the heart contracts. While the pressure is dropping, the hormone **norepinephrine** rises in the bloodstream. Norepinephrine constricts blood vessels and under normal circumstances raises the blood pressure.

Many authorities contend that the rise in norepinephrine after exercise is a safety mechanism in which the body reflexively attempts to maintain proper blood pressure. The stand-still posture after exercise, however, overcomes the action of norepinephrine so the pressure drops anyway. The rise in norepinephrine and drop in blood pressure coupled with a relatively high heart rate represents circulation that is out of kilter. This set of events can be a triggering mechanism for the onset of irregular heartbeats that can lead to sudden death.

The key to avoiding or at least substantially reducing the probability of sudden death after exercise is to keep moving. Walking at a moderate speed for 5 minutes will prevent blood from pooling in the legs because the contracting muscles squeeze the veins, sending more blood back to the heart. The rhythmic contractions of the leg muscles, called the "muscle pump," act as a second heart, significantly assisting it to meet the body's elevated circulatory demand. Another plus for light physical activity during cool-down is that it hastens the removal of lactic acid that has accumulated in the muscles.

Phase Two: Stretching Exercises

The second phase of cool-down calls for the same stretching exercises that were used during the warm-up. Exercisers probably will note that they tolerate stretching more comfortably after exercise, because of the increase in muscle temperature. Stretching at this time helps to prevent muscle soreness, and it provides the exerciser an opportunity to stretch the muscles that have been contracting repeatedly during the performance of exercise. This helps to maintain flexibility of the muscles and joint structures.

Bent leg sit-ups should be added to the routine. Strong abdominal muscles are a postural aid because they provide support for the upper torso. Those who cannot do sit-ups correctly

because of unused and weak abdominals should do modified sit-ups. Correct performance requires that the back be rounded as the participant sits up. Figures 3.12 through 3.13 present some good cool-down exercises.

WALKING FOR HEALTH AND FITNESS

Walking is the natural form of locomotion for human beings. All humans walk unless some form of disability prevents it. For sedentary people, walking is a safe, easy, economical, and convenient way to start exercising. It can be a lead-up activity for more strenuous exercise, or its intensity can be manipulated so it can be the primary or only method of exercise. A well-conceived walking program that includes the appropriate pacing, frequency, duration, and performance techniques can meet health, fitness, and racing objectives.

This text focuses on health and fitness walking and will not cover race walking. Race walking involves a unique style of locomotion that requires instruction, knowledge, skill, and practice. Health and fitness walking rather than competitive walking require few special skills and yet is effective in enhancing fitness and health.

If you become nauseated after exercise, you should continue to walk. If you feel dizzy to the point that walking is not possible nor advisable, it is best to lie down on your back. This position prevents the blood from pooling in your legs because the horizontal position nullifies the force of gravity. The feeling of nausea and subsequent vomiting when people exercise beyond their capacity is another of the body's safety mechanisms. Vomiting kicks up the blood pressure toward normal, and within minutes, you will begin to feel better.

These Shoes Were Made for Walking

Walking is a low-impact activity that can be done indoors or outdoors, in various climatic conditions, and on varying types of terrain. Shoes have been designed specifically for exercise walking for different terrains. Appropriate footwear adds to the enjoyment of walking and reduces the likelihood of incurring a walking-related injury. The following guidelines should help in the selection of proper walking shoes:

1. The shoes should be well padded at the heel to absorb the impact of landing. Women's shoes, particularly, should be well padded in this area because women tend to land with

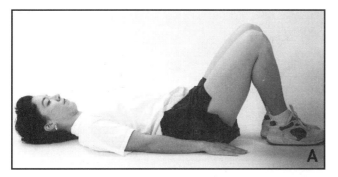

(A) Lie on your back with knees bent and heels close to the buttocks. Extend your arms at your sides.

(B) Curl up with straight arms until your fingertips contact your knees, and return to the starting position. This is a lead-up to more strenuous abdominal exercises. Start with 10 repetitions and progress from there.

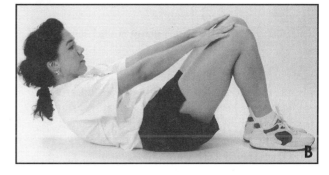

Figure 3.12   Modified Sit-Up.

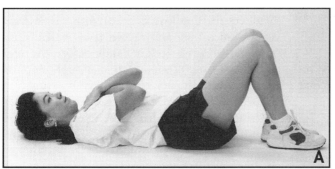

(A) Lie on your back, knees bent, feet close to the buttocks, arms folded across the chest.

(B) Curl up until your shoulder blades lose contact with the floor. Return to the starting position. Start with 10 repetitions, and progress from there.

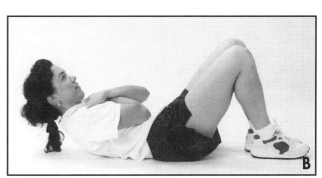

Figure 3.13   Sit-Up.

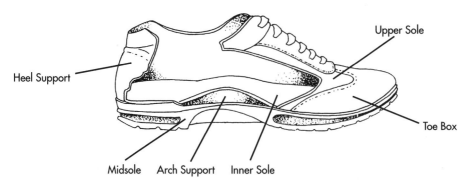

Heel Support

Upper Sole

Toe Box

Midsole   Arch Support   Inner Sole

Figure 3.14   A typical walking shoe.

more force per body weight than men at all walking speeds. The heels on all walking shoes should be 1/2 to 3/4 of an inch higher than the sole.

2. The shoes should fit snugly at the heel and instep (the arched upper part of the foot) and should follow the foot's natural shape.

3. The outer sole should be constructed of durable solid rubber or carbon rubber for long wear. The tread should be designed for good traction.

4. The inner soles should include removable arch supports and heel cups that can be removed after a workout so they can air out and dry.

5. The upper portion of walking shoes should be constructed from leather, synthetic fabrics, or a combination. These materials allow the feet to breathe and provide foot comfort.

6. All walking shoes are relatively lightweight. Unless you are a competitor, you do not have to purchase the lightest shoes on the market, and actually you should not. Foot protection rather than shoe weight is most important for people who walk for health and fitness.

7. Shoes should be selected for function rather than color or fashion.

8. Beginners might do well to purchase their first couple of pairs of walking shoes from a sporting goods store that specializes in sports footwear. Their professional sales people can assist in selection and proper sizing of the shoes.

The Energy Cost of Walking

Walkers do not lose contact with the surface upon which they are traversing. A walker's advancing or striding foot lands before the rear foot leaves the ground. The rear foot supports the weight of the body while the advancing foot is swinging forward. During a brief period, both feet are simultaneously in contact with the ground. At slow speeds, the normal walking gait, with its relaxed arm swing, is an efficient form of locomotion that actually conserves and reduces energy expenditure. To some extent, this is a drawback to the development of physical fitness, but research indicates that walking efficiency decreases and energy expenditure increases as walking speed increases.[15]

The faster you walk, the more calories you burn. This is not the case with jogging, where speed is irrelevant. Jogging a 10-minute mile is much more comfortable, yet burns about the same number of calories as jogging a 6-minute mile.

Table 3.2 provides a comparison of the caloric expenditure for walking at different speeds for selected body weights. This table presents walking speed in miles per hour (mph), and each speed is translated into minutes and seconds to walk 1 mile at that pace. For example, walking at 3.5 mph, the walker would cover the mile distance in 17 minutes and 10 seconds (17:10). If the walker weighs 150 lbs, he or she expends 4.2 kcals/min or 72 kcals per mile (17.17 × 4.2 = 72). Note that seconds must be converted into hundredths of a minute by dividing the number of seconds by 60 (10/60 = .166). Kcals (kilocalories) is the symbol used to denote the caloric value of foods, and this symbol will be used throughout the text.

Table 3.2 indicates that the kcal cost of walking increases significantly at speeds above 3.5 mph. This is primarily because we become less efficient as walking speed rises above 3.5 mph. The differences in kcals expended in walking 5 mph versus 3 mph is 34 kcals per mile for a 150-pound person. If these speeds are maintained for an hour, the difference is 318 kcals.

Body weight also has an impact on energy expenditure for both walking and jogging. Walking at 3.5 mph, a 120-pound person burns 3.4 kcals/minute, while a 210-pound person burns 5.9 kcals/minute. This is a difference of 2.5 kcals/min for every minute walked and a 150-kcal difference for 60 minutes.

The energy expenditure of walking can be increased by swinging the arms vigorously, by swinging hand-held weights, by walking up hills, or any combination of these. A word of caution: Vigorously swinging hand-held weights can result in shoulder soreness or injury. It also might lead to abnormally high blood pressure if the weights are gripped tightly. Vigorously swinging the arms without weight is safer; the difference in caloric expenditure and fitness development will not be significant. Also, ankle weights can distort the natural gait and lead to injury. Hill walking significantly increases energy demand and should be part of the program. Hill walking should be approached cautiously at first, attempting steeper and longer hills as fitness improves, and walking the hills faster. Caloric expenditures at different grades and different speeds are given in Figure 3.15.

The Mechanics of Walking

Walking at 3 mph is considered to be casual walking or strolling. At 4 mph walking progresses to brisk or fitness walking. Walking 5

Table 3.2 Energy Cost of Walking, Kcals/Minute

Body Weight (lbs.)	Walking Speed (mph)						
	2.0 (30 m/m)*	2.5 (24 m/m)	3.0 (20 m/m)	3.5 (17:10 m/m)	4.0 (15 m/m)	4.5 (13:20 m/m)	5.0 (12 m/m)
120	2.3	2.6	3.0	3.4	4.4	5.6	7.2
150	2.8	3.3	3.7	4.2	5.6	7.0	9.0
180	3.4	4.0	4.5	5.0	6.7	8.4	10.8
210	4.0	4.6	5.2	5.9	7.8	9.9	12.6

*m/m = minutes

Note: To find the kcals expended per minute, locate the appropriate body weight and move horizontally until you reach your speed of walking. Kcals expended per minute is located where the two intersect. For example, a 180-lb. person walking at 4 mph would expend 6.7 kcals/min. Kcals per mile would equal 100.5 (15 m/m × 6.7 = 100.5 kcals/m). If this same individual walks at 4 mph for 40 minutes, the kcals expended are 40 × 6.7 = 268 kcals.

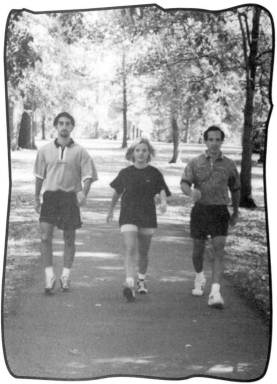

Proper walking posture is erect but relaxed.

mph and faster becomes race pace. The faster one walks, the faster the arms swing. The converse is true as well: Walking speed can be increased by concentrating on swinging the arms rapidly because leg speed tends to follow arm speed. Obviously, walking at 3 mph does not require rapid arm movement, whereas walking at 5 mph does. The purpose in this book is not to produce race walkers but, rather, to provide solid information that will encourage regular participation in health and fitness walking. Rapid speeds are not necessary to enhance health or develop fitness. Vigorous arm swinging, however, is just as important for increasing the energy requirements of walking as it is for increasing speed. Walking at a brisk 4 mph with energetic arm swinging increases the energy cost of walking materially.

Proper walking technique requires an erect, but not stiff posture, in contrast to the incorrect posture of looking down at the walking surface and bending the neck. Instead, the head is erect and scans the road surface with the eyes only. Bending the neck forward to watch where you are stepping will cause you to lean forward. This

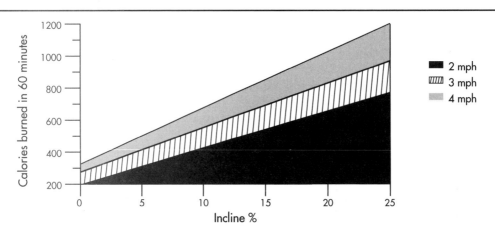

Approximate number of kcal used in an hour by a 150-pound person walking uphill at different speeds on various inclines.

Reprinted with permission from the University of California at Berkeley *Wellness Guide to Lifelong Fitness*, © Health Letter Associates, 1993. For more information, please call 1-800-829-9170.

 Figure 3.15   Kcals used walking uphill.

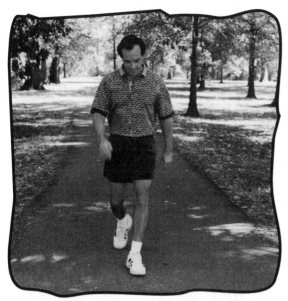

Incorrect walking posture is head and neck forward, eyes looking down.

position strains the lower back, upper back, and neck. It requires the static contraction of extraneous muscles and wastes energy.

The arms should be held with a 90-degree bend at the elbows. The hands should be loosely closed and relaxed. For efficiency, the arms should swing vertically and the hands should travel no higher than the earlobes. The arms are bent at 90 degrees throughout the entire swing. Increasing walking speed is difficult if the arms swing from the shoulders in pendulum style.

In walking, the initial point of contact with the ground is the heel of the foot. This applies to all styles of walking from casual strolling to race walking. As speed increases, foot placement changes. During normal gait walking or strolling, the feet land on either side of an imaginary line that proceeds in the direction of travel as illustrated in Figure 3.16. As speed increases to brisk walking, the stride lengthens and the feet land closer to the imaginary line. In race walking, the feet actually land on the line.

When the heel contacts the ground, the knee should be slightly bent. The landing foot rolls forward, accepting the weight of the body as the rear foot provides a forceful push from the toes. This is repeated rhythmically with every step.

A Summary of Walking Tips

1. Beginners should walk at a comfortable pace.
2. The posture should be erect but not stiff.
3. Arms should be bent at a 90-degree angle at the elbows.
4. Hands should be loosely clenched.
5. Arm swing should be vigorous with the hands traveling no higher than the earlobes. This will increase the caloric expenditure of walking by 5% to 10%.
6. The striding leg lands on the heel and the force rolls up to the toes.
7. The rear foot provides a strong push-off.
8. The arms and legs move contralaterally — the right arm and left leg move forward together, and the left arm and right leg move forward together.
9. The effort can be increased safely by lengthening the distance, increasing the speed,

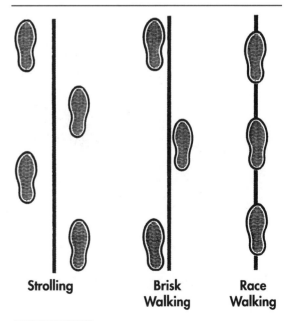

Strolling　　　**Brisk Walking**　　　**Race Walking**

Figure 3.16 Changes in foot placement in various walking speeds.

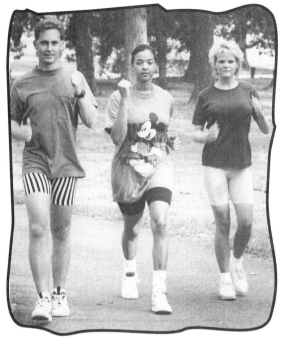

In speed walking or fitness walking, the arms are bent 90 degrees at the elbows and swing vigorously. The hands should not go higher than the earlobes on the upswing.

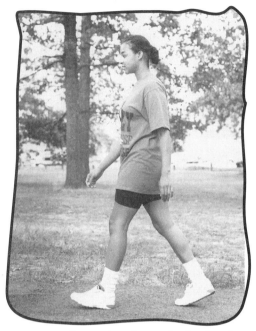

In normal-gaited walking, the heel strike on landing, the knee is bent upon taking the body weight, and the push-off from the toes of the rear foot.

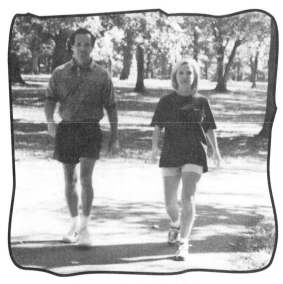

In normal-gaited walking, the arms swing like a pendulum.

swinging the arms vigorously, and walking up hills.

10. Beginning exercisers should walk on alternate days and gradually increase the distance. When you can walk for 30 to 45 minutes without undue fatigue, you can increase the frequency to 4 to 5 days per week. If it meets your objectives, intensity can be increased after satisfying frequency and duration.

JOGGING FOR HEALTH AND FITNESS

Jogging is the activity of choice for millions of Americans. Both fitness and health objectives can be attained expeditiously with a jogging program, and this is part of its appeal. Among the benefits of jogging:

♦ It is one of the best activities for conditioning the cardiorespiratory system, as well as most of the body's largest and most powerful muscles.

- ♦ It is excellent for weight loss and weight maintenance.
- ♦ It is an excellent relaxer and stress reducer.
- ♦ It reduces the risk factors for cardiovascular disease.
- ♦ It reduces susceptibility to many other chronic diseases.
- ♦ It can be performed recreationally, competitively, alone, or with others.

These Shoes Were Made for Jogging

The most important investment a prospective jogger can make is to purchase quality shoes. Proper selection is important because an appropriate, well-fitting pair of shoes can prevent or alleviate blisters, shin splints, and ankle, knee, and hip-joint injuries.

Shoes made especially for jogging have some common characteristics, shown in Figure 3.17. The heel should be about one-half inch higher than the sole, and it should be well padded. The sole should consist of two separate layers. The outer layer should be made of a durable rubberized compound for traction and longevity. The inner layer should be thick and pliable and made of shock-absorbing material. The heel and sole preferably flare out so the impact with the ground can be distributed over a wider area. This is crucial because the jogger's foot hits the ground 600 to 750 times per mile and each foot strike absorbs a force equivalent to three times the body weight. It should come as no surprise that the incidence of stress injuries rises proportionately to the number of miles jogged.

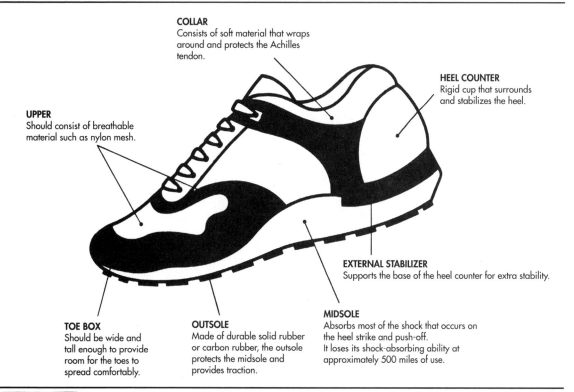

COLLAR
Consists of soft material that wraps around and protects the Achilles tendon.

HEEL COUNTER
Rigid cup that surrounds and stabilizes the heel.

UPPER
Should consist of breathable material such as nylon mesh.

EXTERNAL STABILIZER
Supports the base of the heel counter for extra stability.

TOE BOX
Should be wide and tall enough to provide room for the toes to spread comfortably.

OUTSOLE
Made of durable solid rubber or carbon rubber, the outsole protects the midsole and provides traction.

MIDSOLE
Absorbs most of the shock that occurs on the heel strike and push-off. It loses its shock-absorbing ability at approximately 500 miles of use.

Figure 3.17   Characteristics of a typical jogging shoe.

Flexibility, another characteristic of a good shoe, can be determined by grasping the heel in one hand and the toe in the other and bending it. If it does not bend easily, it is too stiff and inflexible for jogging.

Proper fit is essential. The shoes should be one-half inch longer than the longest toe, and the toe box should allow enough room for the toes to spread. The toe box should be high enough not to pinch the toes. The heel of the foot should fit snugly in the padded heel of the shoe, for maximal support and minimal friction. The shoe should have a good, firm arch support.

When purchasing a pair of shoes, you should wear the same type of sock you will wear when jogging, to minimize errors in sizing. Some attention also should be given to shoe maintenance. It's best to own more than one pair of shoes so they can be rotated from workout to workout. One pair will suffice, however, if they are allowed to dry between workouts.

Shoes should be inspected periodically and discarded if they wear deep into the outer layer. As the shoe wears, the angle of the foot strike changes, producing forces at sites in the legs and hips to which the jogger is unaccustomed. This increases the likelihood of injury.

Of the shock-absorbing qualities of jogging shoes, 30% dissipates at about 500 miles of wear, regardless of price, brand, or type of construction.[16] At that point it is best to replace your jogging shoes.

Jogging shoes should be purchased from a store that specializes in the sale of sports footwear. The professional salespeople will suggest shoes in your price range that are appropriate to your needs.

The Energy Cost of Jogging

The energy cost of jogging for a given body weight is about the same regardless of speed. In fact, the net energy cost of jogging (total kcals used minus kcals that would be used while at rest) is exactly the same. Table 3.3 provides the gross and net kcals used by selected body weights at different speeds. The first line for each weight presents the gross and net kcals per minute, and the second line presents the gross and net kcals per mile.

Note that the net kcals do not change with speed, but the gross kcals change with speeds slightly for the same body weight. An individual weighing 120 pounds uses the same number of

Table 3.3 Gross/Net Kcal Expenditure for Jogging*

Body Weight (lbs.)	MPH Speed (min per mile)	4.0 15.0	5.0 12.0	6.0 10.0	7.0 8.30	8.0 7.30	9.0 6.40	10.0 6.0
120	Kcals (min)	6.5/5.5	7.8/6.9	9.2/8.3	10.8/9.8	12/11.1	13.3/12.4	14.8/13.8
	Kcals (mile)	97/83	94/83	92/83	92/83	90/83	89/83	89/83
150	Kcals (min)	8.1/6.9	9.8/8.7	11.5/10.4	13.4/12.2	15.1/13.9	16.8/15.6	18.5/17.3
	Kcals (mile)	121/104	118/104	115/105	114/104	113/104	112/104	111/104
180	Kcals (min)	9.7/8.3	11.8/10.4	13.8/12.5	16.1/14.7	18.1/16.7	20.1/18.7	22.2/20.8
	Kcals (mile)	146/125	141/125	138/125	137/125	136/125	134/125	133/125
210	Kcals (min)	11.3/9.7	13.8/12.2	16.1/14.6	18.8/17.2	21.1/19.5	23.4/21.9	25.8/24.3
	Kcals (mile)	170/146	165/146	161/146	160/146	158/146	156/146	155/146

* The first number in each set is gross kcals; the second number is net kcals. The first set of numbers for each body weight is kcals per minute for each speed; the second set is kcals per mile for each speed. Example: A 150-lb person jogging at 6 mph will expend 11.5 gross kcals/min; 10.4 net kcals/min; 115 gross kcals/mile; 105 net kcals/mile.

net kcals per mile whether he or she jogs at 4 mph or 8 mph. At 8 mph, the individual will be generating energy at twice the rate expended at 4 mph but will be jogging for only half the time, so the net kcals expended per mile will be the same. The gross expenditure per mile actually decreases as speed increases, but the reduction is insignificant. Joggers can shorten the workout by running faster and still use the same number of kcals per mile, or they can jog slower at a more comfortable rate of speed for a longer time and expend about the same number of total kcals.

The net caloric cost of jogging 1 mile is twice that of walking a mile on level ground at moderate speeds. But at higher rates of walking speed (5 mph or faster), the caloric cost of running 1 mile is only 10% more than walking 1 mile (see Table 3.4). Notice that the net energy expenditure for walking is quite stable up to 3.5 mph. Above this speed, the net kcals increase rapidly so the energy expenditure for walking and jogging come closer together. A 150-pound person walking and jogging at the same speed expends similar amounts of energy on a per-mile basis.

For example, if this 150-pound person walks and jogs at 5 mph, the difference in energy expended per mile is only 10 kcals. Examine Tables 3.3 and 3.4 closely, and compare the two for kcals burned for different body weights and different speeds. Based upon your exercise objectives, the data in these tables might contribute to your selecting the exercise mode that is right for you.

The Mechanics of Jogging

A comfortable erect posture with the head level encourages the correct body alignment for jogging. The eyes should survey the path in front of you for obstacles and irregular terrain, but the neck should not be bent forward. Do not look directly in front of your feet, because this detracts from jogging efficiency and it leads to muscle strain in the neck and lower back if the posture is maintained for some time.

The hands, which are loosely closed, should be carried slightly lower than the elbows for energy conservation and comfort. This posture tends to relax the neck and shoulders. The low hand position mitigates against generation of the powerful pumping action from the arms, but this is not necessary for jogging. Sprinters require power from the arm swing; joggers swing the arms for rhythm and balance. The arms

Table 3.4 Gross/Net Kcal Expenditure for Walking*

Body Weight (lbs.)	MPH Speed (min per mile)	2.0 30	2.5 24	3.0 20	3.5 17:8	4.0 15	4.5 13:20	5.0 12
120	kcals (min)	2.3/1.4	2.6/1.8	3.0/2.1	3.3/2.5	4.4/3.5	5.6/4.7	7.2/6.3
	kcals (mile)	69/42	63/42	59/42	57/42	66/52	75/63	86/75
150	kcals (min)	2.9/1.7	3.3/2.2	3.7/2.6	4.2/3.0	5.5/4.3	7.0/5.9	9.0/7.8
	kcals (mile)	87/52	79/52	74/52	72/52	82/65	93/78	108/94
180	kcals (min)	3.5/2.1	4.0/2.6	4.5/3.2	5.0/3.7	6.6/5.2	8.4/7.1	10.8/9.4
	kcals (mile)	104/63	95/63	89/63	86/63	99/78	112/94	129/113
210	kcals (min)	4.0/2.4	4.6/3.0	5.2/3.7	5.8/4.3	7.7/6.1	9.8/8.3	12.6/11.0
	kcals (mile)	121/173	111/173	104/73	100/73	115/92	131/110	151/132

* The first number in each set is gross kcals; the second number is net kcals. The first set of numbers for each body weight is kcals per minute for each speed; the second set is kcals per mile for each speed. Example: A 150-lb person walking at 3.5 mph will expend 4.2 gross kcals/min; 3.0 net kcals/min; 72 gross kcals/mile; 52 net kcals/mile.

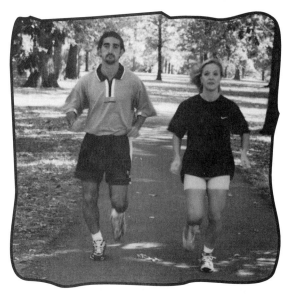

Correct jogging form requires an erect but relaxed posture.

should swing backward and forward and should not cross in front of the body.

The jogging stride should be short and compact, with the foot landing beneath the knee. This aids in keeping the body erect and prevents overstriding. The jogger should land softly on the heel and rock up through the ball of the foot to the toes for the push-off. The body weight transfers from the heel along the outside edge of the foot to the toes. This distributes the impact over a greater surface area and for a longer time, resulting in smooth, energy-efficient locomotion. The landing should be essentially noiseless.

The main difference between walking and jogging is that the body is airborne during each stride while jogging. The airborne or "float phase" accounts for about 30% of the length of stride. The airborne phase represents one of the primary reasons the energy cost of jogging is higher than walking. More energy is required to propel the body into the air with each stride. Overstriding is to be avoided. When the ankle is forward of the knee upon landing, the foot acts as a brake to forward motion. This not only reduces the efficiency of jogging but also puts

stress upon the knee joint, increasing the probability of injury.

Mechanical factors that make jogging such a good aerobic conditioner are the very ones that can produce injury. The fact that joggers are airborne with every step results in a high-impact landing. The ground reaction force when the foot strikes the surface, coupled with the subsequent push-off that propels the body upward, is approximately equal to three times the body weight. Because the average jogger steps between 600 and 750 strides per mile, the knees, hips, and feet absorb the shock of landing that many times. Multiply these values by the number of miles covered in a week, and you can understand the cumulative forces operating on the jogger.

But joggers make a number of biomechanical adjustments that help to dissipate the shock. For example, the flexed position of the knee and ankle when the heel strikes the ground allows the contracting muscles to stabilize the involved joints. In the contracted position, the muscles act as shock absorbers that diffuse the impact of landing. By the time the shock reaches the hip joint, it has been effectively reduced to one-sixth of its original intensity. These adjustments allow joggers to run for many years without serious injuries or premature wear of the joints. Despite this remarkable adaptability, most joggers sustain an injury or two sometime during their many years of jogging. Fortunately, most of these are minor and respond well to rest or treatment.

A Summary of Jogging Tips

1. Sedentary people should ease into jogging, beginning by walking and progressing to a combination of walking and jogging. In the beginning, much more time is spent walking. As fitness improves, walking time is reduced and jogging time is increased until eventually the person will be able to jog for the entire exercise session.

2. The intensity (pace) should be at a low level at first. Frequency and duration should be increased before increasing the intensity.

3. Jogging posture features an erect, but not stiff, body position, with the head level and eyes moving to scan the road ahead.

4. Hands should be slightly lower than the elbows during the arm swing because this promotes relaxation of the neck, shoulders, and jaw.

5. The arms should not swing across the body because this results in rotational sway that decreases efficiency.

6. The correct form is to land on the heel so the large muscles of the legs will absorb the shock of landing.

7. A quality pair of jogging shoes is a must, particularly for running on city streets and sidewalks.

Summary

- A medical exam is desirable prior to starting an exercise program for men 40 years of age and older and for women 50 years of age and older.

- The exerciser's aims and objectives should help to determine how long, how hard, and how often to exercise.

- A warm-up prior to exercise is needed to raise muscle temperature, gently raise the heart rate, and stretch the muscles and joints.

- Static stretching techniques are preferred to dynamic (ballistic) stretching.

- PNF (proprioceptive neuromuscular facilitation) is more effective than static stretching but requires a partner, takes more time, is associated with more pain and muscle stiffness, and is more complex than other forms of stretching.

- Intensity refers to the amount of energy expended per bout of exercise.

- Intensity can be monitored by perceived exertion or target heart rate.

- For the development of fitness, the ACSM recommends an intensity level equal to 55/65% to 90% of the HR max.

- For the development of health, the ACSM recommends moderately intense exercise (walking 3 to 4 mph).

- The Karvonen method for determining target heart rate uses the resting heart rate and cardiac reserve.

- The most common sites for taking the pulse are the radial artery at the wrist and the carotid artery at the side of the neck.

- The ACSM recommends that aerobic exercise be performed three to five times per week to develop physical fitness and preferably all days of the week for improving health.

- Exercise that is too hard, too long, or performed too often can lead to staleness.

- The ACSM recommends that exercise should last a minimum of 30 minutes and be done most days of the week.

- The muscles, systems, and organs used in any given activity are the ones that adapt, and they do so in the specific way in which they are used.

- After exercising, 5 minutes of light activity to prevent the pooling of blood in the veins is imperative (called the cool-down).

- Walking shoes should contain certain features to make walking more enjoyable and safer.

- Walking is a low-impact activity because both feet don't leave the ground simultaneously.

- Walking is an efficient form of locomotion except at the higher speeds. The faster one walks, the more calories one burns.

- The energy expenditure of walking can be increased safely by swinging the arms vigorously and by walking up hills.

- Walking contributes to physical fitness and health.

- Shoes designed for jogging are a must because they are constructed to help dissipate the forces generated on impact with the ground.

- The energy cost of jogging for a given body weight is about the same regardless of speed.

- The net caloric cost of jogging 1 mile is twice that of walking 1 mile on level ground at moderate speeds.

- Overstriding occurs when the ankle is forward of the knee upon landing. It should be avoided because the foot acts as a brake and stresses the knee joint.

- Joggers step between 600 and 750 times per mile.

1. American College of Sports Medicine, *ACSM's Guidelines for Exercise Testing and Prescription* (Baltimore: Williams and Wilkins, 1995).

2. R. J. Barnard et al., "Cardiovascular Responses to Sudden Strenuous Exercise — Heart Rate, Blood Pressure, and ECG," *Journal of Applied Physiology*, 34 (1973), 833.

3. J. E. Kovelaski, L. R. Gurchiek, and D. H. Spriggs, "Musculoskeletal Injuries: Risks, Prevention, and Care," *ACSM's Resource Manual for Guidelines for Exercise Testing and Prescription*, 3d edition, edited by J. L. Roitman (Baltimore: Williams and Wilkins, 1998).

4. ACSM, "The Recommended Quantity and Quality of Exercise for Developing and Maintaining Cardiorespiratory and Muscular Fitness, and Flexibility in Healthy Adults," *Medicine and Science in Sports and Exercise*, 30:6 (1998), 975–991.

5. D. C. Nieman, *Exercise Testing and Prescription A Health — Related Approach* (Mountain View, CA: Mayfield, 1999).

6. D. M. Fredette, "Exercise Recommendations for Flexibility and Range of Motion," *ACSM's Resource Manual for Guidelines for Exercise Testing and Prescription*.

7. ACSM, "The Recommended Quantity and Quality of Exercise."

8. Nieman.

9. R. R. Pate, "Physical Activity and Public Health," *Journal of the American Medical Association*, 273:5 (Feb. 1995), 402–407.

10. M. L. Foss and S. J. Keteyian, *Fox's Physiological Basis for Exercise and Sport* (Boston: WCB McGraw-Hill, 1998).

11. ACSM, "The Recommended Quantity and Quality of Exercise."

12. Ibid.

13. Ibid.

14. I-M Lee et al. "Exercise Intensity and Longevity in Men, The Harvard Alumni Study," *Journal of the American Medical Association*, 273:15 (1995), 1179–1184.

15. E. T. Howley and B. D. Franks, *Health Fitness Instructor's Handbook* (Champaign, IL: Human Kinetics, 1997).

16. T. P White, *The Wellness Guide to Lifelong Fitness* (Rebus, NY: Random House, 1993).

Physiological Adaptations to Walking and Jogging

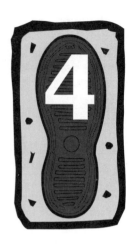

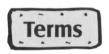

Aerobic

Anaerobic

Anaerobic threshold

Atrophy

Blood pressure

Cardiac output (Q)

Conduction

Convection

Dehydration

Diastolic blood pressure

Disease atrophy

Essential hypertension

Evaporation

Hematocrit

Hyperthermia

Hypothermia

Ischemia

Lactate threshold

Metabolism

Oxygen debt

Oxygen deficit

Radiation

Stroke volume (SV)

Systolic blood pressure

Ventilation

VO$_2$ max

A number of physiological adjustments occur as the body shifts gears from rest to physical exercise. Physical exertion requires prompt physiological and metabolic adaptations to meet the increase in energy demand. These adaptations are differentiated into two categories according to response and effect. The first category, the acute effects, are temporary and occur during and after every bout of exercise. They occur to exercisers regardless of whether they are trained or untrained. Normal physiology and metabolism are regained during the recovery period following the workout. The length of the recovery period varies according to the exerciser's fitness level, the intensity, and the duration of the workout.

The second category, chronic effects (also known as the "training effect") are longlasting and accumulate during exercise performed consistently over weeks, months, and years. The training effects become evident during the first couple of months of exercise, and improvement in fitness continues for many years. Both the acute and chronic effects will be identified and explained in this chapter.

Walking and jogging often are performed outdoors, so it is important to become acquainted with the environmental conditions that increase the risk of outdoor exercise. These will be covered in a fair amount of detail in this chapter.

ACUTE ADAPTATIONS — TEMPORARY EFFECTS

Acute adaptations to walking and jogging are physiological changes that occur during and after a single bout of exercise. We should recognize these adjustments and understand that they are temporary. Some selected acute physiological changes are discussed next.

Heart Rate

The heart's response to walking and jogging is immediate and dynamic. The rate of beating increases with the first few strides and continues to do so until reaching a steady state. Steady state (leveling off of heart rate) occurs only when the intensity of the workout is within the individual's capacity. It represents a period during jogging or fast walking when the body can supply the oxygen demand of the activity on a minute-by-minute basis. This is the essence of an aerobic workout. The term **aerobic** literally means "with oxygen." An activity is aerobic if participants can perform at a comfortable pace (mild to moderately vigorous) so that they can supply the oxygen (O_2) needed during performance ("steady state" exercise). When steady state is achieved, the O_2 demand of exercise and O_2 supplied by the body are in balance.

Steady state cannot be attained for vigorous exercise because the O_2 requirement exceeds the exerciser's ability to supply it while exercising. This type of high-intensity exercise is **anaerobic,** which literally means "without oxygen." Anaerobic exercise can be sustained for only a few seconds. Walking and jogging are aerobic exercises. Sprinting is an anaerobic exercise. High-speed walking and jogging are anaerobic for people who are not trained to perform at these levels.

This text emphasizes the aerobic aspects of walking and jogging because this is an effective and safe approach to enhancing health and improving cardiorespiratory fitness for the majority of adults of all ages.

Aerobic exercises require an increase in blood flow to the exercising muscles. The increase in heart rate with exercise is one of the major mechanisms for accommodating the muscle's demand for blood.

Stroke Volume

Stroke volume (SV) refers to the amount of blood the heart can eject in one beat. The size of the stroke volume depends upon the amount of blood returning to the heart, the dimensions of the systemic pumping chamber (left ventricle), and the force of the contraction. Stroke volume rises linearly; it is correlated positively with increases in workload up to 40% to 60% of capacity and then levels off.[1] From this point on, further increases in blood flow occur as the result of increases in heart rate. The higher stroke volume of trained people represents one of the major differences between them and untrained people and accounts for their ability to sustain endurance activities. Figure 4.1 shows the relationship between heart rate and stroke volume during maximum exercise.

Stroke volume is measured in milliliters (ml) of blood ejected per heartbeat. The average resting and maximum stroke volumes for different levels of training appear in Table 4.1.

Cardiac Output

Cardiac output (Q) represents the amount of blood pumped by the heart in 1 minute. It is the product of heart rate and stroke volume (Q = HR × SV). Cardiac output increases as the intensity of exercise increases. At first it increases because both heart rate and stroke volume increase. Stroke volume levels off when exercise reaches approximately 50% of capacity, so further increases in cardiac output are the result of elevations in heart rate.

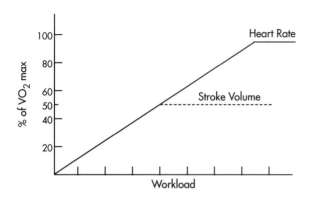

Figure 4.1 Heart rate and stroke volume responses to maximum exercise.

The average value for cardiac output at rest is approximately 4 to 6 liters of blood per minute with values reaching 21 to 25 liters during maximal exercise.[2] Well-conditioned athletes can achieve as much as 40 liters during very high-intensity work. Cardiac output at rest and maximal exercise for untrained, trained, and highly trained individuals appear in Table 4.2.

Table 4.1 Average SV Values At Rest and During Exercise

	Untrained	Trained	Very Highly Trained
At rest	≤70 ml (2.4 oz.)	≤ 90 ml (3 oz)	≥ 130 ml (4.4 oz)
During maximum exertion	≤ 120 ml (4.1 oz.)	≤ 140 ml (4.7 oz)	≥ 200 ml (6.8 oz)

Note: The SV amounts are given in ml, and their equivalent weight in ounces are provided for a better appreciation of the effects of training.

Table 4.2 Average Cardiac Output Values for Untrained, Trained, and Highly Trained People

	Untrained	Trained	Very Highly Trained
At Rest	4 to 6 L	4 to 6 L	4 to 6 L
During Maximum Exertion	16 to 20 L	21 to 25L	34 to 40 L

Blood Flow

The body has the remarkable capacity to shunt blood to tissues that have the most need. For example, blood flow to the working muscles increases during physical activity. This is accomplished by reducing blood flow to other tissues and organs such as the liver, kidneys, and digestive system. In competing for the available blood, the muscles take precedence during physical activity. Blood flow to the digestive system increases after a meal because this represents the greatest area of need. If physical activity occurs immediately after eating, blood is shunted away from the digestive system to the muscles, which slows or temporarily stops digestion depending upon the severity of the exercise. This is one of the main reasons a workout should not begin until at least 1 hour after a meal.

During hot weather, more blood than usual is shunted to the skin to help cool the body. The skin competes with the exercising muscles for the available blood, which results in the muscles receiving slightly less blood than normal. Less blood means less oxygen and nutrients for exercise, so the workout becomes more difficult. This is why exercise in hot weather should be less vigorous and last for a shorter time.

Blood Pressure

Blood pressure is the force exerted by the heart as it pumps blood into the arteries. It is measured in millimeters of mercury (mmHg) with an instrument called a sphygmomanometer. Blood pressure is expressed in two values: systolic and diastolic. The systolic blood pressure is the pressure of the flow of blood when the heart beats. The diastolic blood pressure is the pressure between heartbeats. A typical pressure for a young adult might be 120/70 (read as 120 over 70).

The systolic pressure rises during exercise — a normal and expected response resulting from an increase in cardiac output. Cardiac output increases to supply the blood and oxygen needed by the muscles and the organs (heart and lungs) that support exercise. The blood vessels in these

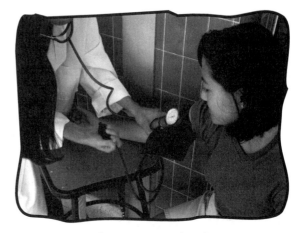

Normal apparatus and technique
for measuring blood pressure.

tissues dilate to accept the extra blood, but their ability to dilate is limited. Because the increase in cardiac output is greater than the stretching ability of the blood vessels, the systolic blood pressure rises. The increase in systolic blood pressure during exercise should not exceed 260 mmHg, as that amount of increase is abnormal and symptomatic of a cardiovascular problem.[3]

The diastolic blood pressure changes little during dynamic or aerobic exercise. The change usually is less than 20 mmHg plus or minus. A rise in the diastolic blood pressure to 115 mmHg is excessive and is considered an abnormal response to exercise.[4]

Blood Volume

Fluid is removed from all areas of the body to produce the perspiration needed to cool the exerciser. Some of this fluid comes from the blood plasma, which reduces blood volume. As a result, the ratio of red blood cells to plasma volume, known as the hematocrit, increases. This increases the viscosity of the blood and inhibits the delivery of oxygen. Viscosity is the thickness of the blood (more solids than liquid), which increases the blood's resistance to flow. The ratio of red blood cells to plasma volume returns to normal as fluids are consumed following the workout.

Respiratory Responses

The average person breathes 12 to 16 times per minute at rest and 40 times per minute during maximal exertion. Ventilation (V), the amount of air inhaled and exhaled per minute, is a product of the frequency of breathing (f) and the volume of air per breath, or tidal volume (TV). At rest, the lungs typically ventilate 5 to 6 liters of air each minute. For example, 14 breaths per minute at 0.4 liter per breath results in a ventilation rate of 5.6 liters of air/minute.

$$\begin{aligned} V &= f \times TV \\ &= 14 \times 0.4 \text{ liters} \\ &= 5.6 \text{ liters} \end{aligned}$$

Ventilation can escalate to 100 liters or more during maximal exertion. Large, well-conditioned athletes move as much as 200 liters per minute.

The movement of large volumes of air from the lungs during exercise places a burden upon the respiratory muscles. The energy cost of breathing at rest represents 1% to 2% of the total oxygen consumed,[5] but during vigorous exercise the cost can increase to 15%.[6] The muscles of the chest wall that expand the rib cage and the muscles of the diaphragm and abdomen require more O_2 to ventilate the lungs during vigorous exercise.

Two respiratory phenomena — side-stitch and second wind — remain mysteries in terms of their etiology. Side-stitch is a pain in the side that can be severe enough to stop activity. Constant pressure applied with both hands at the site of the stitch sometimes alleviates the pain and allows continued activity. Breathing deeply while extending the arms overhead also might provide some relief.

A side-stitch is more likely to occur during jogging, although fast walking can also produce it. No scientific evidence explains the cause or causes of developing a side-stitch, but current opinion indicates that the probable cause is ischemia (diminished blood flow) to the diaphragm or intercostal muscles. The diaphragm is a large dome-shaped muscle that separates the chest cavity from the abdominal cavity. It is the major respiratory muscle responsible for inhalation of air into the lungs.[7] The intercostal muscles, located between the ribs, alternately expand and contract the rib cage for inspiration and expiration of air into and out of the lungs.

"Second wind" is an adaptation in which the perceived effort of exercise seems to become considerably less although the intensity level does not change. The mechanisms involved are not completely understood, but when a person gets a second wind, breathing becomes less labored and experiences a sense of comfort and well-being. It is possibly a result of more efficient circulation to the active tissues or of a more efficient metabolic process."[8] Regardless of the mechanisms, the end result of attaining second wind is that exercise becomes more comfortable.

Metabolic Responses

Metabolism increases with the inception of exercise and continues to do so in direct proportion to increases in exercise intensity. Metabolism can be measured indirectly with appropriate equipment, by the amount of oxygen consumed during exercise on a treadmill, bicycle ergometer, or similar devices. As the intensity of exercise increases steadily, the individual's ability to supply the oxygen needed to keep pace will plateau eventually. This plateau represents the upper limit of endurance and is referred to as maximal oxygen consumption (VO_2 max). Also known as aerobic capacity or cardiorespiratory endurance, it defines a point at which further increases in exercise intensity do not elicit further increases in oxygen consumption. This is depicted in Figure 4.2.

VO_2 **max** represents the body's peak ability to assimilate, deliver, and extract oxygen and is considered to be the best indicator of physical fitness. It is a well-defined exercise endpoint that can be measured and reproduced accurately in

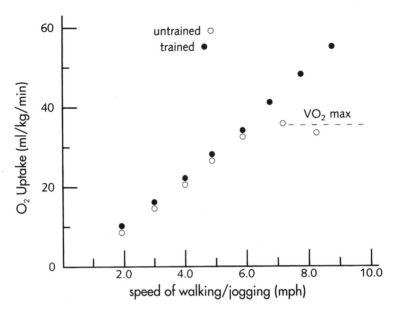

VO_2 max of trained and untrained people.

the laboratory. These procedures are not generally available to the public, but fortunately field tests have been developed that correlate fairly well with the lab tests and may substitute for them. These will be discussed later in this chapter.

Body Size and O_2 Utilization

VO_2 max is measured in liters of oxygen utilized per minute. This absolute value is influenced considerably by body size. Because all body tissues need and use oxygen, larger people take in and use more oxygen both at rest and during exercise. Aerobic capacity, when expressed in liters of oxygen per minute, is not conducive to comparison, as it will yield false results. To eliminate the influence of size, aerobic capacity must be considered in terms of oxygen utilization per unit of body mass. This is accomplished by converting liters of oxygen to milliliters and then dividing by body weight in kilograms.

For example, a 220-pound person uses 4.5 liters of O_2 per minute during maximum exertion, and a 143-pound person's capacity is 3.5 liters of O_2 per minute. From these data, the larger person seems to be more aerobically fit because of a greater capacity to use oxygen. Observe what occurs, though, when these values are corrected for body size. Divide body weight in pounds by 2.2 to convert to kilograms:

$$\frac{220 \text{ lbs.}}{2.2 \text{ kg.}} = 100 \text{ kg}$$

Now convert liters of O_2 per minute (LO_2/min) to milliliters of O_2 per minute by multiplying LO_2/min by 1000 (4.5 LO_2/min $\times$ 1000 = 4500 ml O_2/min). Or you can just move the decimal point three places to the right to accomplish the same result.

Person A
4.5 LO_2/min = 4500 ml. O_2/min
4500 ml. O_2/min $\div$ 100 kg (220 lbs) = 45 ml. O_2/kg/min.

Person B

3.5 LO$_2$/min = 3500 ml. O$_2$/min

3500 ml. O$_2$/min ÷ 65 kg (143 lbs) = 54 ml. O$_2$/kg/min.

From this example, the lighter person clearly can transport, extract, and use more oxygen per unit of body mass than the larger person and is better equipped to perform endurance activities. VO$_2$ max values expressed in ml O$_2$/kg/min. range from the mid-20s in sedentary older people to 94, which is the highest documented value recorded so far. This enormous capacity belongs to an extremely well-conditioned male cross-country skier. The highest value recorded for female athletes is 74, also by a cross-country skier. College-age females typically have values in the upper 30s to low 40s.

Effects of Gender on VO$_2$ max

Gender differences in aerobic capacity become evident after puberty, when females exhibit lower VO$_2$ values. The difference is attributed to smaller heart size per unit of body weight, less oxygen-carrying capacity because of lower blood hemoglobin concentration, less muscle tissue, and more body fat.[9] The sexes overlap considerably regarding aerobic capacity, though. World-class females competing in endurance events are aerobically superior to most males, but they have lower values than world-class male competitors. The differences between males and females are probably a combination of true physiological limitations and cultural restraints that have been placed upon females regarding endurance training and competition. The influence of culture and biology on female performance eventually will become clearer as more females train and compete during the next decade.

Effects of Age on VO$_2$ max

The decline in VO$_2$ max seems to parallel the functional losses as people age. Less than 50% of this loss is attributable to the aging process, and the remainder to an inactive lifestyle. Maximum heart rate, cardiac output, stroke volume, and metabolism decrease during the adult years. Body composition changes as muscle tissue is lost, thereby decreasing the body's energy-producing machinery. An increase in fat tissue is an impediment to physical performance.[10] Breathing capacity decreases as the thoracic cage (chest) loses some of its elasticity, caused by weakened intercostal muscles (muscles between the ribs), increased residual volume (air remaining in the lungs after expiration), and increased rigidity of lung structures. These changes can be delayed significantly by consistent participation in exercise and physical activity.[11]

O$_2$ Deficit/O$_2$ Debt

When exercise begins, a short interval of time is needed for the body to adjust to the increased oxygen demand. This period when the oxygen demand of exercise exceeds the body's transport capability is referred to as the **oxygen deficit**, as illustrated in Figure 4.3.

A second phenomenon — **oxygen debt** — occurs during both aerobic and anaerobic exercise (see Figure 4.3). Oxygen debt refers to the amount of oxygen consumed during the exercise recovery period above that normally consumed while at rest. It is measured at the end of exercise and includes the oxygen deficit.[12] During anaerobic exercise, the body cannot supply all the oxygen needed, resulting in a deficiency between supply and demand that must be repaid at the end of exercise. A 10-second sprint or running up two or three flights of stairs elevates the heart rate and ventilation. Both persist for a few moments following the activity before gradually returning to resting levels. The extra oxygen consumed during this interval represents the oxygen debt. Aerobic exercise also produces an oxygen debt that may be entirely due to the oxygen deficit, particularly in low-intensity exercise. Aerobic exercise in excess of 50% of the aerobic capacity will produce lactic acid and a further increase in oxygen debt.

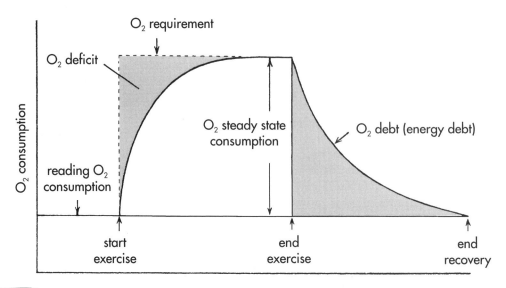

Figure 4.3 The O₂ deficit and O₂ debt.

CHRONIC ADAPTATIONS — TRAINING EFFECTS

Chronic adaptations, also referred to as long-term effects, are the physiological and psychological changes that result from training. These changes represent the training effect that is gradually developed after repeated bouts of exercise.

Heart Rate

A few months of fast walking or jogging will produce a decrease in the resting heart rate (RHR) by 10 to 25 beats per minute. The decrease in resting heart rate is accompanied by a decline in exercise heart rate for a given workload. For example, a jogging speed that elicits a heart rate of 150 beats per minute prior to training might invoke a heart rate of 125 beats per minute after a few months of training. A period of 5 to 6 months will lower the submaximal exercise heart rate by 20 to 40 beats per minute. Also, the exercise heart rate returns to the resting level more rapidly as physical fitness improves.

The importance of lowered resting and exercise heart rates is that this allows more time for filling the ventricles of the heart with blood to be pumped to all of the body's tissues and more time for delivering oxygen and nutrients to the heart muscle. The delivery of these substances occurs during diastole (resting phase of the heart cycle) because relaxation of the heart muscle allows the coronary vessels to open up and receive the blood that they need. Training substantially prolongs the heart's diastolic phase with the net result that the heart operates more efficiently and with longer periods of rest.

Stroke Volume

Stroke volume and heart rate are inversely related at rest; as stroke volume increases, heart rate decreases. The heart rate at rest and for a given workload is lower because of the heart's enhanced ability to pump more blood per beat. This is accomplished because of more complete filling of the left ventricle combined with an increase in the contractile strength of its muscular walls, resulting in a more powerful contraction and greater emptying of the blood in the chamber. This stronger, more efficient heart is capable of meeting circulatory challenges with less beats at rest and during submaximum exercise. Training significantly increases the maximum stroke volume. In fact, the single greatest difference in the performance of untrained people and endurance-trained people is the size of the stroke volume.

Cardiac Output

Post-training cardiac output increases considerably during maximum exercise, but it changes little during rest or submaximal work, primarily because the trained individual is able to extract more oxygen from the blood. The oxygen concentration in arterial blood is essentially unchanged, but the extraction rate (a-vO$_2$ difference) might increase significantly. With training, the a-vO$_2$ difference increases, resulting in more oxygen being used, as reflected by less oxygen in the venous blood. The increase in cardiac output during maximum exercise represents another major difference between untrained and endurance-trained people.

Blood Pressure

High blood pressure is a major risk factor for heart disease. To lower the risk, elevated blood pressure has to be reduced. The vast majority of high blood pressure (90% to 95% of the cases) is categorized as **essential hypertension**. *Essential* is a medical term meaning the cause is unknown. *Hypertension* is the medical term for high blood pressure. Although essential hypertension has no cure, it can be treated and controlled successfully.[13]

Exercise is one of the important behavioral factors that has the potential to prevent and treat established hypertension. After examining years of research evidence, the American College of Sports Medicine has drawn the following conclusions regarding the relationship between exercise and high blood pressure:[14]

1. Endurance exercise training reduces blood pressure by about 10 mmHg (millimeters of mercury) in individuals who have mild hypertension (140/90 mmHg to 180/105 mmHg).

2. Lower intensity exercise, 40% to 70% of aerobic capacity, seems to reduce blood pressure as much or more than higher-intensity exercise.

3. Physically active and aerobically fit hypertensives have substantially lower death rates than physically inactive hypertensives. Aerobic exercise tends to nullify many of the harmful effects of hypertension.

Scientists have yet to identify all of the mechanisms through which exercise lowers blood pressure, but the following probably are involved:

1. Norepinephrine is a vasoconstrictor that clamps down on the blood vessels, increases resistance to blood flow, and raises blood pressure. Exercise lowers the level of this hormone in the blood, reduces resistance to blood flow, and lowers blood pressure.

2. Exercise likely increases vasodilator substances that dilate or open up blood vessels, decreasing resistance to blood flow.

3. Exercise stimulates the kidneys to reduce the salt level in the blood, which in turn lowers the blood pressure.

4. Exercise contributes to weight loss, which is one of the most effective means to lower blood pressure.

Blood Volume

Blood volume increases with endurance training. The volume change occurs from a significant increase in the amount of plasma (the liquid portion of the blood) and a lesser increase in blood solids (primarily, the number of red blood cells). The increase in plasma volume versus red blood cells is disproportionate. The greater increase in plasma volume results in less viscous blood that is thinner (more watery). This is an important adaptation to training because thinner blood can be circulated more efficiently and with less resistance.

A trained person's red-cell count usually is below average, so the individual could appear to be anemic. In reality, trained people have a higher absolute number of red blood cells than untrained people, but on a relative basis, because of the expanded plasma volume, the numbers appear to be low. The average hematocrit (ratio of red blood cells to plasma volume) of the general public is 40% to 50%. Males have slightly higher values (more red blood cells per unit of blood) than females.

The lower hematocrit of trained people not only is an important adaptation for endurance performance but also represents a healthy change. The ideal hematocrit for running a marathon is about 50%, but for health it probably is closer to 40% for men and 35% for women.[15]

Heart Volume

The heart reacts to persistent walking or jogging in much the same manner as the other muscles of the body do. It becomes stronger and often, larger. The volume as well as the weight of the heart increases with endurance training. Bed rest produces the opposite effect; the heart shrinks in size.

In the not-so-distant past, exercise-induced changes in the heart were considered to be pathological. The term "athlete's heart" was assigned to describe the cardiac hypertrophy (heart enlargement) seen in many athletes, the connotation that such a heart was harmful to health and longevity. Today, the medical community accepts these changes as normal responses to endurance training that have no long-term detrimental effects. In fact, maintaining such a heart for as long as possible would be beneficial. Six months of inactivity following a training program will reduce heart weight and size to pretraining levels. The **atrophy** associated with inactivity is unavoidable.

Respiratory Responses

Some training-induced adaptations also occur in the respiratory system. The muscles that support breathing improve in both strength and endurance. This increases the amount of air that can be expired after a maximum inspiration (vital capacity) and decreases the amount of air remaining in the lungs (residual volume). As a result of training, **ventilation** decreases slightly for a given workload and increases significantly during maximum exercise. This indicates an improvement in the efficiency of the system. The depth of each breath (tidal volume) also increases during vigorous exercise.

Training increases blood flow in the lungs. In the sitting or standing position, many of the pulmonary capillaries in the upper regions of the lungs close down because gravity pulls blood down to the lower portions of the lungs. Exercise forces blood into the upper lobes and creates a greater surface area for the diffusion of oxygen from the alveoli (air sacs) to the pulmonary blood. This perfusion of the upper lobes of the lungs is improved with training.

Metabolic Responses

Endurance training improves aerobic capacity (VO_2 max) by 5% to 30%.[16] The magnitude of the increase depends primarily upon the initial level of fitness. Those who are the least fit make the most improvement simply because they are farthest away from their genetic potential.

Fitness gains come rather quickly during the first few months of training, and further increases occur in smaller increments as fitness improves until VO_2 max reaches its peak, after 6 months to 2 years of training.

Improvement in VO_2 max results from a combination of physiological adaptations.

1. The number and size of mitochondria increase. The mitochondria (often referred to as the cells' powerhouse) are organelles within the cells that utilize oxygen to produce the ATP the muscles need. ATP (adenosine

triphosphate) is a high-energy compound that provides the fuel the body uses.

2. Enzymes located within the mitochondria that accelerate the chemical reactions needed for the production of ATP are increased. These increases in the mitochondria and their enzymes produce greater amounts of energy and improvement in physical fitness.

3. Maximal cardiac output and local blood supply in the exercising muscles increase.

4. The exercising muscles extract more oxygen from the blood. At rest, the arteries carry approximately 20 ml O^2 per 100 ml of blood. The veins carry about 14 ml O^2 per 100 ml of blood. When the oxygen value in the veins is subtracted from the oxygen value in the arteries, it yields the amount of oxygen the body uses. This value is termed the arterial-venous oxygen difference (a–vO_2 diff), and at rest it is equal to 6 ml O_2/100 ml blood. Because exercise increases the body's need for oxygen, the extraction rate increases and the a-vO_2 difference widens. Training increases the a-vO_2 difference during maximum exercise but might not increase it at rest or during submaximum exercise.

Effect of Aging on the Aerobic System

Aerobic capacity decreases with age, but it decreases more slowly for people who are physically fit. Researchers at San Diego State University studied the effect of exercise on 15 men who walked, jogged, swam, and cycled 3 to 4 days per week for 23 years.[17] The men averaged 45 years of age at the start of the study and 68 years at the 23-year mark. Their VO_2 max declined 13% during 23 years, equivalent to a 5% reduction per decade in VO_2 max, compared to sedentary adults whose expected loss per decade approximates 9% to 15%.[18]

Physically fit 60-year-olds have an aerobic capacity equal to unfit people who are 35 years younger. Physical training delays the deterioration

often associated with aging. Current evidence suggests that at least 50% of the changes attributed to aging (weight gain, stooped posture, loss of muscle mass and strength, loss of energy) actually are attributable to a decline in physical activity. These physical changes are characterized by the term **disease atrophy**. The average loss in VO_2 max as people age is a gradual but systematic 1% per year.

The researchers concluded that the 13% loss in VO_2 max for the exercise group represented a true effect of aging. If the aging effect (13% decline) is factored out of the decline of the nonexercisers, two-thirds of their decrease in VO_2 max results from inactivity rather than aging.

This important long-term study has provided evidence to support what many exercisers and researchers already knew by logical deduction and anecdotal evidence: that physical training delays the deterioration of aerobic capacity at least until people reach their 60s.

Effect of Inherited Factors

Aerobic capacity is finite. Each of us is endowed with an aerobic potential limited by our heredity. A small percentage of people inherit the potential to achieve amazing feats of endurance, as exemplified by performances in marathons, ultramarathons, Iron Man triathalons, cross-country runs lasting weeks or months, and long-distance bike races. Although most of us are in the average category for aerobic capacity, we can achieve our potential with endurance training.

Researchers have attempted to quantify the influence of heredity as a component of VO_2 max. How much of the variability seen among people in VO_2 max comes from inherited factors? Although this line of inquiry is yet to be fully resolved, the differences observed among identical twins, fraternal twins, and other siblings have provided some clues. The best available evidence suggests that the genetic component represents a range of 25% to 40% of the known factors regarding the achievable VO_2 max for any individual.[19] Individuals who have inherited superior cardiorespiratory endowment have the physical structure to benefit maximally from training and could become national or world-class performers if they train diligently and intelligently. Those who are endowed to a lesser extent (the majority of people) also can benefit from training. They do not have the foundation to become high-level competitors, but they can train to their potential and enjoy their own accomplishments.

Anaerobic Threshold — Lactate Threshold

Even though VO_2 max reaches a peak early in the training program, aerobic performance continues to improve for many years with harder and continued training. The question, then, is, how can physical performance continue to improve after VO_2 max has leveled off? This question can be answered with an example. Let us assume that a female jogger has achieved her aerobic potential of 54 ml/kg/min after 2 years of regular training. At this point she is able to jog a 5-mile course at 38 ml/kg/min, or 70% of her aerobic capacity. After 2 more years of vigorous training (VO_2 max still at 54 ml/kg/min), she now is able to sustain a 47 ml/kg/min pace for the same distance, or 88% of her aerobic capacity. The past 2 years of training have permitted her to use more oxygen, thereby sustaining a faster pace for the course without dipping materially into the anaerobic fuel systems that produce lactic acid and oxygen debt.

The point during exercise at which blood lactate suddenly begins to increase is defined as the **anaerobic threshold** or **lactate threshold**. Training moves the anaerobic threshold closer to the VO_2 max, allowing people to exercise at a higher percentage of their capacity before lactic acid accumulates to the point at which it begins to interfere with muscle contraction and physical performance. Two people with the same VO_2 max will perform differently in an endurance event if one has an anaerobic threshold substantially higher than the other.

DECONDITIONING — LOSING THE TRAINING EFFECT

Deconditioning takes place when training is discontinued or significantly reduced. E. F. Coyle investigated the physiological changes that accompany detraining, as well as the approximate timetable of their occurrence.[20] The subjects in this study had been actively training for 10 years. They abandoned training for 84 days (12 weeks) so Coyle could observe and measure the changes that took place. Coyle noted that some systems of the body showed the effects of detraining rapidly, while others reacted more slowly. Stroke volume declined substantially in the first 12 days. As expected, the decline was accompanied by a significant reduction in aerobic capacity, which declined 16% by the 56th day of the deconditioning period. The oxidative enzyme level in the muscles had dropped 40% by the end of 8 weeks. By the end of the detraining period, however, the capillary density of the muscles had declined by only 7% below the trained state, and mitochondrial enzymes remained 50% higher than those of the sedentary control subjects. As a result of detraining, both heart muscle mass and blood volume also decreased.

WALKING/JOGGING IN VARIOUS CLIMATIC CONDITIONS

Human beings are compelled to function in a variety of environmental conditions. People live and work in frigid, temperate, and tropical zones, at sea level and at high altitudes, and have adapted and learned to tolerate extremes in temperature. In cold weather, body temperature can be maintained by putting on more clothes or by increasing the body's production of heat through physical movement or shivering. In hot environments, heat is lost through sweating, increasing the blood flow to the skin, or by wearing as little clothing as the law and culture will allow.

Hot Weather

Humans are homeotherms (meaning "same heat"), capable of maintaining the constant internal temperature necessary to support life-sustaining processes such as cellular metabolism, oxygen transport, and muscular contraction. We exist within a relatively narrow band of internal temperature, ranging from 97 to 99 degrees F., although our temperature can (and often does) rise to 104 degrees during exercise.

Body temperatures that rise above 106 degrees, if not rapidly reduced, often result in cellular deterioration, permanent brain damage, and death. Temperatures below 93 degrees slow metabolism to the extent that unconsciousness and cardiac arrhythmias (disturbances of normal heart rhythm that can be fatal) are likely.

The body produces heat as a byproduct of metabolism. Physical activities increase metabolism significantly, generating more heat than normal. If heat is not dissipated effectively, **hyperthermia** can result in illness and possible death. Hyperthermia is abnormally high body temperature. Heat exhaustion is a serious condition but not an imminent threat to life. It is characterized by dizziness, fainting, rapid pulse, and cool skin. Treatment includes immediate cessation of activity and moving to a cool, shady place. The victim is placed in a reclining position and given cool fluids to drink.

Heat stroke, the most severe of the heat-induced illnesses, is a medical emergency and a threat to life. Symptoms include high temperature (approximately 106 degrees F or above) and dry skin caused when sweating stops. These symptoms are accompanied by some or all of the following: delirium, convulsions, and loss of consciousness. Early warning signs include chills, nausea, headache, and general weakness. Victims of heat stroke should be rushed to the nearest hospital immediately for treatment.

Mechanisms of Heat Loss and Heat Transfer

Heat is lost from the body by conduction, radiation, convection, and evaporation of sweat.

Conduction, convection, and radiation are mechanisms responsible for heat transfer. The weather conditions determine through these mechanisms whether walkers and joggers lose or gain heat. Evaporation of sweat is a true heat loss mechanism because the transfer of heat can travel only in one direction — from the body to the environment.

Conduction   **Conduction** occurs when two objects, one cooler than the other, come into direct physical contact. The greater the difference in temperature between the objects, the greater is the transfer of heat. If you enter an air-conditioned room from outdoors on a summer day and sit in a cool leather chair, you will lose heat through contact with the cooler chair.

Conductive heat loss occurs even more rapidly in water. Water is a conductor. It absorbs several thousand times more heat than does air at the same temperature. This is the reason that sitting at the poolside is more comfortable than sitting in the pool, even if the air and water temperatures are equal.

Convection   Heat loss by **convection** occurs when a gas or liquid that is cooler than the body moves across the skin. If the gas or liquid is warmer than skin temperature, the body will accept heat rather than lose it.

Convective heat loss from the body to the environment increases if a cool breeze is blowing, whether it be induced naturally or caused by an electric fan. Convective heat loss accelerates if the body is immersed in cool water. Swimming is more effective than floating for heat loss because of the flow of water over the body. When one participates in water activities, convective heat loss is augmented by conductive heat loss. Heat-loss and heat-transfer mechanisms do not function in isolation; they often work together to rid the body of heat.

Radiation   Heat is lost through **radiation** because humans, animals, and inanimate objects constantly emit heat by electromagnetic waves to cooler objects in the environment. This occurs without physical contact between objects. Heat is simply transferred on a temperature gradient from warmer objects to cooler ones.

Heat loss by radiation is very effective when the air temperature (ambient temperature) is well below skin temperature. This is one of the major reasons that outdoor exercise in cool weather is better tolerated than the same exercise in hot weather. Temperatures in the upper 80s and 90s will probably result in heat gain by radiation.

Evaporation The primary way by which heat is lost is **evaporation** of sweat. This process is most effective when the humidity is low. High humidity significantly impairs the evaporative process because the air is already saturated and cannot accept much more moisture. High temperature and high humidity impede heat loss. Under these conditions, adjusting the intensity and duration of exercise or moving indoors where the climate can be controlled might be beneficial.

Heat loss by evaporation occurs only when sweat on the skin surface is vaporized or converted to a gas. The conversion of liquid to gas at the skin level requires heat supplied by the body. Beads of sweat that roll off the body do not contribute to the cooling process. Only the sweat that evaporates does.

Exercise in hot and humid conditions forces the body to divert more blood than usual from the working muscles to the skin in an effort to carry the heat accumulating in the deeper recesses to the outer shell. The net result is that the exercising muscles are deprived of a full complement of blood and cannot work as long or as hard. Exercise, therefore, is more difficult in hot and humid weather.

Heat loss by evaporation is seriously impeded when participants wear nonporous garments such as rubberized and plastic exercise suits. These garments encourage sweating, but their nonporous nature does not allow sweat to evaporate. This practice is dangerous because it easily can result in heat build-up and **dehydration,** leading to heat-stress illnesses. Exercisers

should dress for hot-weather exercise by wearing shorts and a porous top. A mesh, baseball-type cap is optional; it is effective in blocking the absorption of radiant heat when exercising in the middle of the day, because the sun's rays are vertical. When exercising during cooler parts of the day and when the sun is not shining, a cap makes no difference.

Guidelines for Walking and Jogging in Hot Weather

Guidelines for exercising in heat and humidity have been developed for road races. These can be applied to any strenuous physical activity performed outdoors during warm weather. Outdoor conditions for exercise are safe when any combination of heat and humidity fall into the "safe" category as defined in Figure 4.4. The figure includes instructions on how to use the chart. Caution should be used when the temperature and humidity exceed these values. People who are trained and heat acclimated can continue to exercise at higher temperatures and humidities, but they should take precautions to prevent heat-related illness.

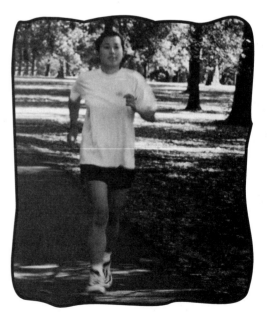

Warm weather jogging clothing
should be lightweight to promote cooling.

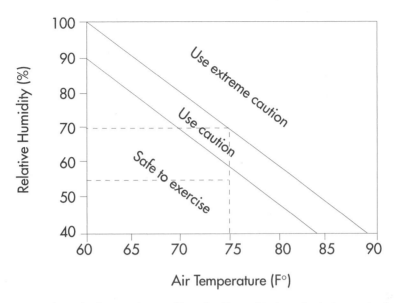

Note: There is an inverse relationship between heat and humidity. To use this chart plot the intersection between the heat and humidity. For example: If the temperature is 75 degrees and the humidity is 70% the intersect lands between "caution" and "extreme caution." But a temperature of 75 degrees is safe if the humidity is 55%.

Figure 4.4 Guidelines for exercise in heat and humidity.

Notice the relationship between temperature and humidity in the figure. The higher the percent humidity, the lower the temperature must be to exercise safely. Conversely, the lower the humidity, the higher the temperature can be for exercise to be safe.

The keys to exercising without incident in hot weather are to acclimate to the heat and to maintain the body's normal fluid level. The major consequence of dehydration (excessive fluid loss) is a reduction in blood volume.[21] This results in sluggish circulation that decreases the delivery of oxygen to the exercising muscles. Second, lowered blood volume results in less blood that can be sent to the skin to remove the heat generated by exercise. If too much of the blood volume is lost, sweating will stop and the body temperature will rise, leading to heat-stress illness. Heat illness is a serious problem that can be avoided by following a few guidelines designed to preserve the body's fluid level:

1. Hyperhydration — pre-exercise:[22]

   a. The exerciser should remain fully hydrated between days of exercise. This involves drinking fluids often, even when you are not thirsty. Waiting to drink until you become thirsty means that dehydration is taking place.

   b. The exerciser should drink at least 16 ounces of water, preferably more, 15 to 20 minutes prior to a workout.

2. Fluid replacement during exercise. The primary reason for drinking during exercise is to maintain body water stores so sweating can continue:

   a. Water is the preferred fluid to drink when exercise lasts less than 90 minutes. Water exits the stomach rapidly and moves to the tissues that need it.

b. Urine production slows during exercise because fluid is used to produce sweat.

c. A beverage containing salt and sugar is preferred if exercise lasts longer than 90 minutes (for example, during marathons, long-distance cycling, and ultra-distance running events and triathalons).

d. The exerciser should drink 8 ounces every 15 minutes during exercise.

3. Post-exercise fluid replacement:

a. Post-exercise fluid should be cold (45° to 55° F) because this will absorb some of the body's heat, which helps cool the exerciser, and cold water leaves the stomach more rapidly than tap water, thereby meeting tissue needs sooner.

b. After exercise the exerciser should drink one pint (16 ounces) of water for each pound of body weight that was lost during exercise.

c. The exerciser should avoid alcoholic beverages and caffeinated beverages because these stimulate the production of urine. The body needs to retain all ingested fluids for the purpose of rehydration.

d. Exercisers can opt to drink fluids that contain salt and sugar. Commercial sports drinks are appropriate. In addition, they taste good, which encourages exercisers to drink more. This counteracts the tendency of most people to drink less water than they need.

4. Because 95% of the weight lost during exercise is fluid, weight loss becomes a good indicator of the amount of fluid loss. For estimating fluid loss:

a. Weigh yourself in the nude before and after exercise.

b. Towel off sweat completely after exercise and then weigh yourself.

Each pound of weight loss represents about 1 pint of fluid loss. The exerciser should drink that and more after exercise.

5. Other considerations:

a. The exercise program can be modified by

(1) working out during cooler times of day,

(2) choosing shady routes where water is available,

(3) slowing the pace and/or shortening the duration of exercise on particularly oppressive days,

(4) wearing light, loose, porous clothing to facilitate the evaporation of sweat.

b. Salt tablets are taboo. They are a stomach irritant, they attract fluid to the gut, they sometimes pass through the digestive system undissolved, and they can perforate the stomach lining.

c. For the average bout, the exerciser need not worry about depleting potassium or make a special effort to replace it. To reduce potassium stores, exercise has to be prolonged, produce profuse sweating, and occur over a number of consecutive days. Daily consumption of fresh fruits and vegetables, as suggested by food consumption guidelines, is all that is needed.

Cold Weather

Problems related to exercise in cold weather include frostbite and hypothermia (abnormally low body temperature). Frostbite can lead to permanent damage or loss of a body part from gangrene. Frostbite can be prevented by adequately protecting exposed areas such as fingers, nose, ears, facial skin, and toes. The exerciser should wear gloves, preferably mittens or thick socks, to protect the fingers, hands and wrists. A stocking cap is recommended because blood vessels in the scalp do not constrict effectively, so a significant amount of heat is lost if the person does not wear a head covering, and a stocking cap hat can be pulled down to protect the ears.

In very cold or windy weather, surgical or ski masks and scarves will keep the face warm and will moisten and warm inhaled air. All exposed or poorly protected flesh is vulnerable to frostbite when the temperature is low and the wind chill is high. Table 4.3 can be used as a safety guide for working and exercising in cold, windy weather. Notice the relationship between the temperature and wind speed. A temperature of 40° F feels like 16° F if the wind is blowing at 25 mph.

People often develop a hacking cough for a minute or two after physical exertion in cold weather. This is normal and should not cause alarm. Very cold, dry air may not be fully moistened when it is inhaled rapidly and in large volumes during exercise. This causes the lining of the throat to dry out. When the person stops exercising, the respiratory rate slows and the volume of inhaled air decreases, allowing enough

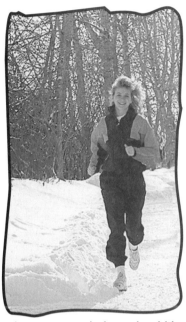

Cold weather exercise clothing should be layered to trap and retain body heat.

Table 4.3 Wind Chill Index

Wind Speed (mph)	Actual Thermometer Reading (°F)											
	50	40	30	20	10	0	−10	−20	−30	−40	−50	−60
	Equivalent Temperature (°F)											
Calm	50	40	30	20	10	0	−10	−20	−30	−40	−50	−60
5	48	37	27	16	6	−5	−15	−26	−36	−47	−57	−68
10	40	28	16	4	−9	−21	−33	−46	−58	−70	−83	−95
15	36	22	9	−5	−18	−36	−45	−58	−72	−85	−99	−112
20	32	18	4	−10	−25	−39	−53	−67	−82	−96	−110	−124
25	30	16	0	−15	−29	−44	−59	−74	−88	−104	−118	−133
30	28	13	−2	−18	−33	−48	−63	−79	−94	−109	−125	−140
35	27	11	−4	−20	−35	−49	−67	−82	−98	−113	−129	−145
40*	26	10	−6	−21	−37	−53	−69	−85	−100	−116	−132	−148

Little danger (for properly clothed person)   Increasing danger — cover up fully (hands, ears, face, head)   Great danger — exercise indoors

* Wind speeds higher than 40 mph have little additional effect.
From *Physiology of Fitness*, by B. J. Sharkey (Champaign, IL: Human Kinetics Books, 1990). Reprinted by permission.

time for the body to fully moisturize it. Coughing stops within a couple of minutes as the linings are remoistened.

Of the problems associated with outdoor activity in cold weather, **hypothermia** is the most severe. It occurs when body heat is lost faster than it can be produced. This can be life-threatening. Heat is lost primarily by convection because of the large difference between the skin and the temperature of the air.[23]

Exercise in cold weather requires insulating layers of clothing to preserve normal body heat. Without this protection, body heat is lost quickly because of the large temperature gradient between the skin and the environment. In addition to the insulating qualities of layers of clothing, a layer or two can be discarded if you get too hot.

Hypothermia can occur even if the air temperature is above freezing. For instance, the rate of heat loss for any temperature is influenced by wind velocity. Wind velocity increases the amount

of cold air molecules that come in contact with the skin. The more cold molecules, the more effective is the heat loss. The speed of walking or jogging into the wind must be added to the speed of the wind chill.

The exerciser should wear enough clothing to stay warm but not so much as to induce profuse sweating. The amount of clothing appropriate for outdoor activities depends upon the experience that comes from participating in cold weather conditions. Clothing that becomes wet with sweat loses its insulating qualities and becomes a conductor of heat, moving it from the body quickly and potentially endangering the exerciser.

ASSESSING CARDIORESPIRATORY ENDURANCE

Aerobic capacity (VO_2 max) is measured quite accurately in the laboratory with a motor-driven treadmill or bicycle ergometer along with gas collection and analysis systems. This equipment is expensive and requires those doing the testing to have considerable expertise. In addition, only one person at a time can be tested, so the investment in time is sizable.

These procedures are inappropriate for large groups. Therefore, investigators have attempted to find economical substitutes that would yield accurate results. Three field tests have been selected in lieu of laboratory tests. They correlate quite well with the laboratory tests and are easier to administer.

Walking Tests

The most used walking tests are the Rockport and the 3-mile walking tests.

Rockport Fitness Walking Test*

The Rockport test estimates aerobic capacity based on the variables of age, gender, time

If you exercise or work outdoors in cold weather, you may want to wear polypropylene undergarments. Polypropylene is designed to whisk perspiration from the skin so evaporative cooling will not rob heat from the body. You should wear a warm outer garment, preferably made of wool, over this material. If it is windy, you should wear a breatheable windbreaker as the outer layer. If you follow the guidelines for activity in hot and cold weather, you usually can participate quite comfortably all year long.

*Rockport provides a series of 20-week walking-for-fitness programs based on results of the walking test. These can be obtained for a nominal fee by sending a request to Rockport Fitness Walking Test, 72 Howe St. Marlboro, MA, 01752.

required to walk 1 mile, and the heart rate achieved at the end of the test. The course should be flat and premeasured, preferably a 440-yard track. A stopwatch or a watch with a secondhand is required. Steps in taking the test are as follows:

1. Warm up for 5 to 10 minutes before taking the test. Preparation for the test should consist of a 1/4 mile walk followed by stretching exercises.

2. During the test, walk at a brisk pace and cover 1 mile as rapidly as possible.

3. Take your pulse rate immediately after the test. Count the heart rate for 15 seconds and multiply by 4 to get beats per minute.

4. Record the rate on the chart on the following pages (Figures 4.5 and 4.6) that is appropriate for your age and gender. Draw a vertical line through your time and a horizontal line through your heart rate. The point where the lines intersect determines your fitness level.

These charts are designed to tell you how fit you are compared with other individuals of your age and gender. For example, if your coordinates place you in the "above average" section of the chart, you are in better shape than the average person in your category.

The charts are based on weights of 170 pounds for men and 125 pounds for women. If you weigh substantially more, your relative cardiovascular fitness level will be slightly overestimated. If you weigh substantially less, your relative cardiovascular level will be slightly underestimated.

3-Mile Walking Test

The 3-mile walking test is a test to fatigue. No running is allowed. The duration of this test and the fact that it demands a maximum effort (walking the distance as quickly as possible) requires you to train at least 6 weeks before attempting it. Students attain their best scores when they first are allowed two practice trials walking the distance. This experience enables

them to find the pace that will result in the fastest time within their fitness capacity. Some suggestions for taking the test are the following:

1. Walk at an even pace, but attempt the fastest pace you can maintain for the entire distance.

2. Avoid starting out too fast. If you do, you will run out of energy too soon.

3. Rest the day before and the day after the test.

4. Eat a predominantly carbohydrate meal (pasta, rice, potatoes, pancakes) that is low in fat. Select foods that have given you no digestive problems in the past. Eat approximately 2 to 3 hours before the test.

5. Drink plenty of liquids the day of the test. Water, Gatorade™, and fruit juices diluted with half water are appropriate.

6. Warm up before the test. About 5 to 6 minutes of walking followed by stretching exercises will suffice.

7. Cool down after the test by walking at a slower pace for 5 to 6 minutes, and do the same stretching exercises as you performed in the warm-up period.

The test is best administered on a running track 1/4 mile long; 12 full laps around will complete the test. After finishing the test, record your time and compare it with the numbers listed in Table 4.4 to determine your fitness level. For example, if a 19-year old female walks the 3 miles in 41 minutes and 28 seconds (41:28), her fitness level is "Fair."

Jogging/Running Test

The best test for jogging/running is the 1.5-mile run test.

1.5-Mile Run Test

The 1.5 mile run has been correlated highly with treadmill tests in the measurement of aerobic capacity.[24] It has the following advantages over laboratory testing:

1. A number of people can be tested at the same time.

20 to 29 Year-Old Males

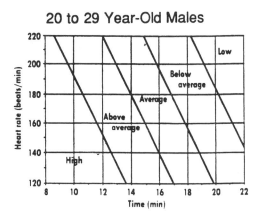

30 to 39 Year-Old Males

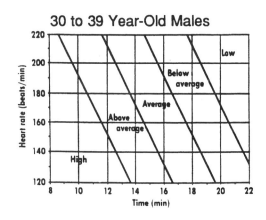

40 to 49 Year-Old Males

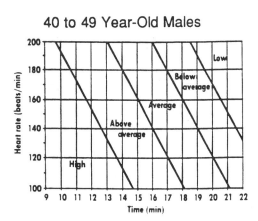

50 to 59 Year-Old Males

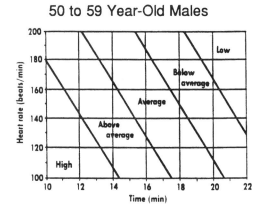

60 Year-Old and Older Males

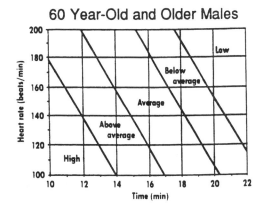

Figure 4.5 Charts for Rockport Walking Test (males).

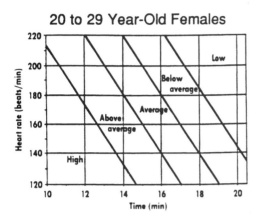

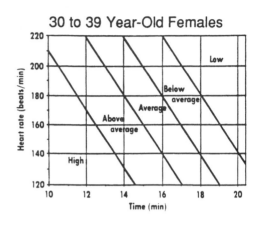

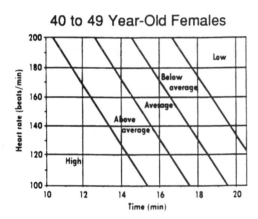

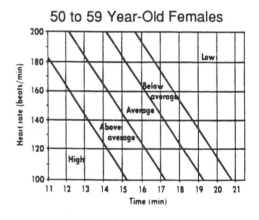

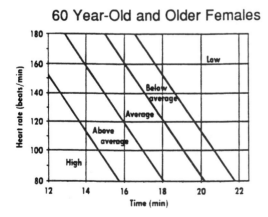

Figure 4.6 Charts for Rockport Walking Test (females).

Table 4.4 Level of Aerobic Fitness — 3-Mile Walking Test

Fitness Category	13–19 Yr		20–29 Yr		30–39 Yr	
	Male	Female	Male	Female	Male	Female
Excellent	<33:00	<35:00	<34:00	<36:00	<35:00	<37:50
Good	33–37:30	35–39:30	34–38:30	36–40:30	35–40:00	37:30–42:00
Fair	37:31–41:00	39:31–43:00	38:31–42:00	40:31–44:00	40:01–44:30	42:01–46:30
Poor	41:01–45:00	43:01–47:00	42:01–46:00	44:01–48:00	44:31–49:00	46:31–51:00
Very Poor	>45:00	>47:00	>46:00	>48:00	>49:00	>51:00

< = Less than; > = greater than

From *Wellness Concepts and Applications* by D. Anspaugh, M. Hamrick, and F. Rosato (St. Louis: Mosby, 1994). Reprinted by permission.

2. The test is easy to administer.

3. The only equipment needed is a measured course and a stopwatch.

The validity and accuracy of the 1.5-mile test can be increased by allowing the testees an opportunity to have several practice trials over the test course, spaced over a week or 10 days. Thus, each subject becomes familiar with the course and with the pace required to produce an optimal score. After several practice trials, each testee attempts to run the course in the fastest possible time within his/her capacity. The most valid results are attained when they make an all-out effort.

The time required to cover the distance represents the score earned. Walking is allowed if the person needs to rest but, of course, it will detract from the score, as it adds time to cover the distance. Table 4.5 translates the time taken to cover the distance into one's estimated aerobic capacity (VO_2 max). After obtaining this value, Table 4.6 is consulted for placement into a fitness category.

For example, a 22-year-old female covers the 1.5-mile distance in 13:20 min. Table 4.5 indicates that she has an estimated VO_2 max of 37 ml/kg/min. Table 4.6 indicates that 37 ml/kg/min falls in the "fair" category but note that the average VO_2 max of females is 15% to 20% lower than that of males. Therefore, to assess this female's fitness level correctly, you must shift one

Table 4.5 Estimate of Aerobic Capacity

Time (in minutes and seconds)	Estimated VO_2 max (in ml/kg/min)
7:30 or less	75
7:31 – 8:00	72
8:01 – 8:30	67
8:31 – 9:00	62
9:01 – 9:30	58
9:31 – 10:00	55
10:01 – 10:30	52
10:31 – 11:00	49
11:01 – 11:30	46
11:31 – 12:00	44
12:01 – 12:30	41
12:31 – 13:00	39
13:01 – 13:30	37
13:31 – 14:00	36
14:01 – 14:30	34
14:31 – 15:00	33
15:01 – 15:30	31
15:31 – 16:00	30
16:01 – 16:30	28
16:31 – 17:00	27
17:01 – 17:30	26
17:31 – 18:00	25

Adapted from "A Means of Assessing Maximal Oxygen Intake," by K. H. Cooper, *Journal of the American Medical Association*, 203 (1968), 201–204. Reprinted by permission.

Table 4.6 Fitness Levels for the 1.5-Mile Jog/Run Test

Age Group (yrs)	High	Good	Average	Fair	Poor
10–19	Above 66	57–66	47–56	38–46	Below 38
20–29	Above 62	53–62	43–52	33–42	Below 33
30–39	Above 58	49–58	39–48	30–38	Below 30
40–49	Above 54	45–54	36–44	26–35	Below 26
50–59	Above 50	42–50	34–41	24–33	Below 24
60–69	Above 46	39–46	31–38	22–30	Below 22
70–79	Above 42	36–42	28–35	20–27	Below 20

Note: The average maximal O_2 uptake of females is 15% to 20% lower than that of males. To find the appropriate category for females, locate the score in the above table and shift one category to the left (the "Average" category for males is the "Good" category for females).

Adapted from *Training for Sport and Activity,* by Jack H. Wilmore (Boston: Allyn and Bacon, 1982). Reprinted by permission.

category to the left so she moves from "fair" to "average." No adjustment is needed in Table 4.6 to assess the fitness level of males correctly.

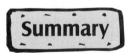

Summary

- The acute adaptations to exercise refer to the physiological changes that occur during and after a single bout of exercise.
- Heart rate and stroke volume rise linearly for exercise of increasing intensity, but stroke volume levels off at approximately 50% of maximum capacity.
- Cardiac output increases during maximum exercise as the result of training.
- The body shunts blood to areas of greatest need — to the muscles during exercise, to the digestive system after a meal, and so on.
- The systolic blood pressure rises during exercise. This is a normal response because of the rise in cardiac output.
- Viscosity of the blood increases during heavy exercise of prolonged duration.

- The energy cost of breathing during rest is about 1% to 2% of the oxygen consumed, but during vigorous exercise the cost could increase to 15%.
- Aerobic capacity (VO_2 max) is the body's peak ability to assimilate, deliver, and extract oxygen for physical work.
- Males generally have higher aerobic capacities than females.
- VO_2 max decreases with age, but age per se is responsible for less than 50% of the decline. Inactivity is responsible for most of the loss.
- Training reduces the resting heart rate and increases the resting and maximum stroke volume.
- Lower intensity exercise, 40% to 70% of VO_2 max, reduces the resting blood pressure for most people by about 10 mmHg.
- Training reduces viscosity of the blood by increasing the plasma volume.
- Heart volume increases with aerobic training.
- Aerobic capacity can be improved by 5% to 30% with aerobic training.

- Inherited factors are responsible for approximately 25% to 40% of a person's achieved aerobic capacity.

- The body systems decondition at various rates when training ceases.

- The body loses heat by conduction, convection, radiation, and evaporation.

- The keys to exercising safely in high heat and humidity are to acclimate to the heat and to be adequately hydrated.

- The most common cold-related exercise injury is frostbite; the most serious cold-weather injury is hypothermia.

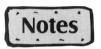

1. E. T. Howley and B. D. Franks, *Health Fitness Instructor's Handbook* (Champaign, IL: Human Kinetics, 1997).

2. D. C. Nieman, *Exercise Testing and Prescription: A Health-Related Approach* (Mountain View, CA: Mayfield, 1999).

3. ACSM, *ACSM's Guidelines for Exercise Testing and Prescription* (Baltimore: Williams and Wilkins, 1995).

4. Ibid.

5. H. A. de Vries and T. J. Housh, *Physiology of Exercise* (Madison, WI: WCB Brown and Benchmark, 1994).

6. W. D. McArdle, F. I. Katch, and V. L. Katch, *Exercise Physiology* (Philadelphia: Lea and Febiger, 1991).

7. M. L. Foss, and S. J. Keteyian, *Fox's Physiological Basis for Exercise and Sport* (Boston: WCB/McGraw-Hill, 1998).

8. J. H. Wilmore and D. L. Costill, *Training for Sport and Activity* (Dubuque, IA: Wm. C. Brown, 1988).

9. R. A. Roberts and S. O. Roberts, *Exercise Physiology, Exercise, Performance, and Clinical Applications* (St. Louis: Mosby, 1997).

10. ACSM Position Stand, "Exercise and Physical Activity for Older Adults" *Medicine and Science in Sports and Exercise*, 30:6 (1998), 992–1008.

11. M. H. Williams, *Lifetime Fitness and Wellness*, (Madison, WI: CB Brown and Benchmark, 1996).

12. Howley and Franks.

13. American Heart Association, *Heart and Stroke Statistical Update — 1997* (Dallas: American Heart Association, 1997).

14. ACSM Position Stand, "Physical Activity, Physical Fitness and Hypertension," *Medicine and Science in Sports and Exercise*, 25:10 (1993), i–x.

15. "What's the Ideal Hematocrit?" *Physician and Sportsmedicine*, 18:8 (Aug. 1990), 35.

16. ACSM Position Stand, "The Recommended Quantity and Quality of Exercise for Developing and Maintaining Cardiorespiratory and Muscular Fitness, and Flexibility in Healthy Adults," *Medicine and Science in Sports and Exercise*, 30:6 (1998), 975–991.

17. F. W. Kasch et al., "The Effects of Physical Activity and Inactivity on Aerobic Power in Older Men (A Longitudinal Study)," *Physician and Sportsmedicine*, 18:4 (April 1990), 73.

18. ACSM Position Stand, 1998.

19. S. N. Blair, "Changes in Physical Fitness and All-Cause Mortality," *Journal of the American Medical Association*, 273:14 (1995), 1093–1098.

20. E. F. Coyle et al., "Effects of Detraining on Responses to Submaximal Exercise," *Journal of Applied Physiology*, 59 (1985), 853.

21. T. D. Noaks, "Dehydration During Exercise: What are the Real Dangers?" *Journal of Clinical Sports Medicine*, 5 (1995), 123–128.

22. ACSM's Guidelines, 1995.

23. T. E. Bernard, "Environmental Considerations: Heat and Cold," in *ACSM's Resource Manual for Guidelines for Exercise Testing and Prescription*.

24. Cooper, p. 38.

Reducing the Risk of Cardiovascular Disease Through Exercise

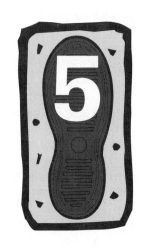

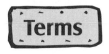

Arterioles
Atherosclerosis
Blood plasma
Cardiovascular
   diseases
Catecholamines
Coronary heart
   disease
Diastolic pressure
Essential hypertension
Folic acid
HDL
Hemoglobin
Homocysteine
Hypertension
Insulin
LDL
Lipoproteins
Lp(a)
Menopause
Morbidity
Mortality

Obesity
Peripheral vascular
   resistance
Serum cholesterol
Subclinical disease
Systolic pressure
Vasoconstrictors

The health benefits associated with walking and jogging, as well as other aerobic exercises, have been researched systematically during the last couple of decades. Evidence supporting health enhancement through consistent participation in physical exercise has been accumulating steadily.

This chapter focuses on the effect of exercise in preventing, delaying, and, to a lesser extent, treating coronary heart disease. To this end, the emphasis is on the modifying effect that exercise has on the risk factors for coronary heart disease.

CARDIOVASCULAR DISEASES

Cardiovascular diseases — diseases of the heart and blood vessels — comprise the leading causes of death in the United States. They are responsible for approximately 39% of the total number of deaths that occur annually.[1] In the United States, 57 million people have one or more forms of cardiovascular disease, nearly 1 million of whom die each year. The leading form of cardiovascular disease, claiming nearly 500,000 lives annually, is **coronary heart disease.** This is the classic type of heart attack that occurs when obstructions (blood clots) or spasms (constricture of coronary vessels) disrupt the flow of blood to a portion of the heart muscle. The site of obstruction or spasm determines the extent of muscle damage. Heart attacks of any magnitude result in irreversible injury and death of the heart muscle. The dead muscle forms scar tissue that no longer contributes to the heart's ability to pump blood. After a heart attack, the heart becomes a less efficient pump. If the attack is massive and causes extensive damage, the heart and its host will die.

Atherosclerosis is the primary cause of coronary heart disease. It is the process in which fatty substances, cholesterol, calcium, fibrin, and cellular debris form plaques that obstruct the flow of blood. If unchecked, plaques continue to enlarge until the arterial channels narrow significantly, creating the environment for blood clots or spasms to occur at these sites of disease. If blood flow is completely impeded, a heart attack will occur and muscle tissue damage will follow (see Figures 5.1 and 5.2).

RISK FACTORS FOR HEART DISEASE

Although most heart attacks occur later in the life cycle (55% after the age of 65) the processes responsible for them begin quite early, often before adolescence. These processes, referred to as cardiovascular risk factors, were identified in the landmark Framingham Heart Disease Study, which began in 1949 and continues today. The

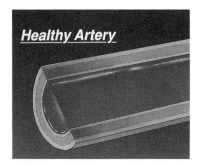 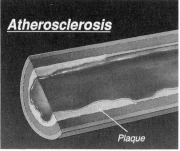 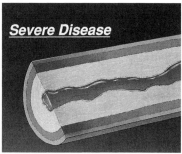

From *Heart of a Healthy Life*. Courtesy of the American Heart Association, © 1992.

Figure 5.1   Plaque build-up at various stages of atherosclerosis.

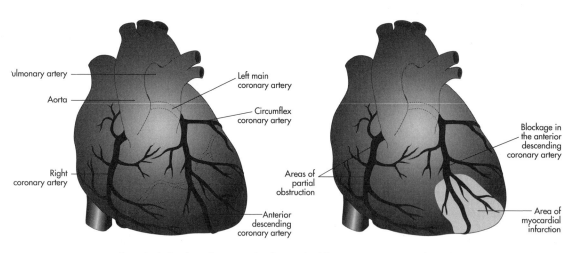

From *Principles and Labs for Physical Fitness and Wellness*, 5th ed. by W. W. K. Hoeger (Englewood, CO: Morton Publishing, 1999).

Figure 5.2   Heart attack caused by a blood clot.

risk factors are either genetic or lifestyle behaviors that increase the probability of premature illness and death from coronary heart disease. The American Heart Association (AHA) has categorized the risk factors as those that cannot be changed, those that can be changed, and other contributing factors.

Risk Factors That Cannot be Changed

Major risk factors that cannot be changed are increasing age, male gender, and heredity.

Age

The statistical probability that a person will die from heart disease increases with advancing age. Although all forms of cardiovascular disease contribute to the death rate, coronary heart disease is responsible for the majority of these.[2] Nonpharmocological (no medicines) approaches featuring exercise, proper nutrition, abstaining from tobacco, and other health promoting lifestyle behaviors substantially lower the risk at any stage of life.

Male Gender

Men are, and have been, the primary candidates for heart disease. An alarming trend has surfaced in recent years though, **morbidity** (the sick rate in a population) and **mortality** (the death rate in a population) have been increasing steadily in premenopausal women. The prime contributor is cigarette smoking, and when it is coupled with taking oral contraceptives, the risk increases substantially.

Coronary heart disease is the leading cause of death and disability among women, accounting for almost 250,000 deaths annually.[3] Normally, premenopausal women are unlikely candidates for heart disease unless they have a family history plus one or more of the other risk factors for the disease. Prior to **menopause** (permanent stoppage of the menstrual cycle) women are at less risk than men because estrogen, the female sex hormone, protects the coronary arteries from premature disease. Also, women have a more favorable blood-fat ratio that protects the arteries from atherosclerosis. Vulnerability to heart disease for women increases after menopause because estrogen production decreases and then stops, and blood-fat ratios change so they resemble the masculine profile. By her 70s, a woman's risk is comparable to that of a man of the same age.

Heredity

Children whose parents have heart disease or atherosclerosis have an increased tendency to develop these problems themselves. A family history of heart disease is confirmed when (a) a father or first-degree male relatives (grandfather or brother) has had a clinically diagnosed heart attack or dies of heart disease prior to 55 years of age, and (b) a mother or first-degree female relative (grandmother or sister) has had a clinically diagnosed heart attack or dies of heart disease prior to 65 years of age.[4]

Risk Factors That Can be Changed

Major risk factors that can be changed are cigarette smoking, high blood pressure, elevated serum cholesterol, physical inactivity and obesity. Other contributing factors are diabetes, and stress.

Cigarette Smoking

Many medical researchers consider cigarette smoking to be the most potent of the preventable risk factors associated with chronic illness and premature death. It is directly responsible for 419,000 deaths from all causes in the United States. Smoking accounts for 30% of all deaths from cancer and 30% of all cardiovascular deaths.[5]

In the decade of the 1960s, 50% of the adult males in the U.S. were smokers. Today, only 25.5% are smokers.[6] During this time, though, smoking among women declined little, and 23% of U.S. women continue to smoke. Smoking is responsible for almost half of all heart attacks in women prior to 55 years of age. Rather than quit, many women have elected to switch to cigarettes that are low in tars and nicotine in an effort to reduce the risk. The evidence indicates that this practice does not materially affect the risk.[7]

According to federal government statistics, smoking is on the rise among teenagers of both sexes. Estimates indicate that 3,000 new teenagers begin smoking every day. Currently, 20% of White teenagers smoke, while 5% of Black teenagers smoke.[8]

Harmful Products in Cigarette Smoke Nicotine, poisonous gasses such as carbon monoxide, tars, and chemical additives to enhance flavor and taste are the harmful substances in cigarette smoke.

Nicotine is a powerful addictive stimulant that has profound effects on the cardiovascular system. It contributes to spasms of the coronary blood vessels, increases the oxygen requirement of the heart at rest and during physical exertion, constricts small blood vessels leading to a rise in blood pressure, and causes irregular heartbeats.

Carbon monoxide is a noxious gas that is a byproduct of the combustion of tobacco products. It displaces oxygen in the bloodstream because **hemoglobin** (a protein pigment transported by red cells that attaches to and carries oxygen) has a much greater affinity for carbon monoxide than oxygen. As a result, the reduced oxygen-carrying capacity of the blood is partially responsible for shortness of breath upon mild physical exertion.

The effects of cigarette smoking are insidious. Some effects appear immediately, and others take years to develop. The medical profession measures the dangers associated with cigarette smoking in pack-years. Pack-years are determined by the number of packs smoked per day multiplied by the number of years smoked. For example, smoking one pack per day for 25 years equals 25 pack-years. Smoking 1½ packs per day for 25 years equals 37.5 pack years. The more years accumulated, the more likely the smoker will be to exhibit smoking-related diseases. Twenty-five years represent a typical threshold for such diseases to manifest themselves.

Passive Smoke and Smokeless Tobacco Products Passive smoke (also called involuntary, secondhand, or environmental smoking) involves inhaling the smoke of others. Those who breathe secondhand smoke have increased risk of premature illness and death. Estimates show that 35,000 to 60,000 nonsmokers die annually of heart disease because of exposure to secondhand smoke, and another 3000 die of lung cancer.[9] Inhaling secondhand smoke has a dose-response relationship with developing smoking-related illnesses. The greater the exposure, the greater is the risk. Children of smoking parents have a higher incidence of influenza, bronchitis, asthma, pneumonia, and the common cold.

In recent years, smokeless tobacco products (chews, plugs, and dips) have become increasingly popular with high school and college males. These products pose another threat. Nicotine is just as addictive and just as harmful when it is delivered through the oral cavity as it is when delivered through the lungs. The effects of carbon monoxide are eliminated from smokeless tobacco products because these are not combustible, but users of smokeless tobacco trade less risk of lung cancer for greater risk of oral cancer. The incidence of oral cancer is 50 times higher among users than among nonusers.[10]

Quitting the Habit Smoking is an extremely difficult habit to break. Success requires overcoming the addiction to nicotine while simultaneously dealing with the psychological dependence on smoking. The latter might be more of a challenge than the former. The person overcomes the nicotine addiction within the first couple of weeks after quitting, but the psychological and social cues remain for years. Breaking this dependence requires reeducation and changes in behavior.

Situations and circumstances that acted as smoking triggers in the past must be dealt with in future encounters. Smokers often light up reflexively in the presence of certain cues. Cues to smoke might be a cup of coffee or an alcoholic drink, the end of a meal, talking on the telephone, situations that produce anxiety or tension, parties, and other social gatherings. The ties between these cues and smoking behavior are difficult to break.

Complicating the desire to quit, particularly among young women, is the fear of gaining weight. Cigarette smoking is, to some extent, a weight-control technique because it is a stimulant that increases metabolism, speeds food through the digestive tract (thereby decreasing the time for absorption of calories and nutrients), and is an appetite suppressant. Cigarette smokers as a group are about 7 pounds lighter than nonsmokers. But smokers tend to deposit more fat in the abdomen and upper body, which increases the risk for heart attack, stroke, diabetes, and some forms of cancer.

Stop-smoking approaches include professional counseling, nicotine patches, nicotine chewing gum, hypnosis, artificial cigarettes, acupuncture, and aversive conditioning. The 1-year success rates for these techniques range from 10% to 40%.

Millions of Americans have quit smoking. The number of adult smokers today is half that of the 1960s. Many of the quitters did so on their own. At this point, the most effective approaches to quitting smoking seem to feature personal and group counseling, a combination of methods and techniques, and supplementary self-help materials.[11]

Exercise offers another option. When people get hooked on the exercise habit, they often disconnect from the smoking habit. Smoking is a

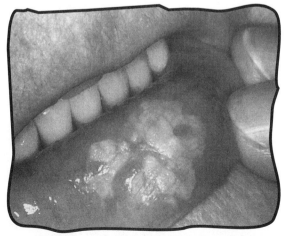

Smokeless tobacco was the cause of this squamous cell carcinoma on the lower lip.

drawback to exercise performance, and it limits the health gains that can be achieved with exercise. Table 5.1 lists some of the physiological changes over time after quitting smoking.

High Blood Pressure

Blood pressure is recorded in millimeters of mercury (mmHg). It is the combined force that circulating blood exerts against the artery walls plus the resistance to blood flow by the arteries. Pressure is created as the heart contracts and pumps blood into the arteries. The smallest arteries (the arterioles) offer resistance to blood flow. If the resistance is consistently high, the pressure increases and remains high. **Hypertension** is the medical term for high blood pressure.

Hypertension has no overt symptoms. It is a silent disease that can be detected only by a blood pressure screening test. Blood pressure consists of two components:

1. **Systolic pressure** represents the maximum pressure of blood flow in the arteries when the heart contracts.

2. **Diastolic pressure** represents the minimum pressure of blood flow in the arteries between heartbeats.

Blood pressure is read as the systolic over the diastolic pressure. A reading of 140/90 or greater is considered to be hypertensive. A blood pressure of 100/60 is considered to be the lowest level of normal; however, some people with lower values function normally and are free of disease. A low normal reading is highly desirable. Table 5.2 classifies blood pressure from normal to hypertension.

Approximately 50 million Americans have blood pressure above 140/90. The causes of 90% to 95% of these cases are unknown. This type of hypertension is called "essential," which is a medical term that means "of unknown origin or cause." Although **essential hypertension** cannot be cured, it can be treated and, usually, controlled.

Longstanding uncontrolled or poorly controlled hypertension has an adverse effect on the heart. It increases its workload so the heart enlarges in response to the strain. Because the blood pressure is consistently high, the heart does not get enough rest. As a result, the heart's muscle fibers become overstretched and progressively lose their ability to rebound. The end result is that the force of contraction weakens and the heart becomes an inefficient pump. If intervention strategies are not enacted early in the process, the heart will suffer irreversible damage. Hypertension also has a detrimental effect on the arteries and accelerates the atherosclerotic process.

Prevention techniques include maintaining recommended body weight, restricting dietary salt, ingesting adequate calcium and potassium, and engaging in voluntary relaxation and exercise.

Treatment of hypertension consists of the same strategies used in prevention, with the addition of medication if these lifestyle changes fail to normalize the blood pressure.

Salt is composed of 40% sodium and 60% chloride. Sodium is the real culprit in salt, as it is associated with rising blood pressure. It does this by encouraging the body to retain fluid so that the **blood plasma** (the liquid portion of the blood) expands. The extra blood imposes a burden on the heart, which must pump blood with more force to circulate it through the arteries.

Daily salt intake should be reduced to a maximum of one-and-one quarter teaspoon; this

Table 5.1 Expected Body Changes That Occur After Smoking Cessation

Time	Changes
20 minutes	♦ Blood pressure and heart rate drop to normal values. ♦ Temperature of hands and feet return to normal.
8 hours	♦ Carbon monoxide in the blood returns to normal.
24 hours	♦ Risk of heart attack begins to decrease.
48 hours	♦ Nerve endings regenerate. ♦ Senses of taste and smell improve.
2 weeks to 3 months	♦ Circulation improves. ♦ Lung function improves by 30%. ♦ Exercise is easier to perform.
1 to 9 months	♦ Coughing and sinus congestion decrease. ♦ Lungs become clearer, with less mucous. ♦ Respiratory infection is less likely. ♦ Energy level increases. ♦ Shortness of breath is not as pronounced.
1 year	♦ The risk of coronary heart disease is half that of a smoker.
5 years	♦ Lung cancer death rate decreases. ♦ Stroke risk is reduced to that of a nonsmoker 5 to 15 years after quitting. ♦ Risk of cancer of the mouth, throat, and esophagus is half that of a nonsmoker.
10 years	♦ Lung cancer death rate is one-half to that of a nonsmoker. ♦ Risk of cancer of the mouth, throat, esophagus, bladder, kidney, and pancreas decreases.
15 years	♦ Risk of coronary heart disease is equal to that of a nonsmoker. ♦ Lung cancer risk is lower but not as low as that of a nonsmoker — in fact, the risk may never get to that point.

Adapted from "Incentives To Quit," *Your Health Network*, 2:1 (First Quarter, 1994), 4.

Table 5.2 Standards for Classification of Blood Pressure for Adults Age 18 Years and Older

Category	Systolic (mmHg)	Diastolic (mmHg)
Normal	< 130	< 85
High Normal	130–139	85–89
Hypertension		
Stage 1 (Mild)	140–159	90–99
Stage 2 (Moderate)	160–179	100–109
Stage 3 (Severe)	180–209	110–119
Stage 4 (Very Severe)	≥ 210	≥ 120

From National Institutes of Health, *The Fifth Report of the Joint National Committee on Detection, Evaluation and Treatment of High Blood Pressure* (Washington, DC: U.S. Dept. of Health and Human Services, January, 1993) NIH Publication No. 93–1088.

translates into less than ½ teaspoon of sodium, or about 2.4 grams.[12] Most of the sodium consumed in the United States comes from processed foods. Of the remainder, 15% comes from using the salt shaker, and another 10% occurs naturally in food.[13] Foods that are heavily laden in salt are frozen dinners, frozen pizza, processed meats (such as bacon, ham, hotdogs), processed American-style cheese, canned and dried soups, canned meats, beans, tomato sauce, most restaurant food, and fast foods. The U.S. Surgeon General, the National Academy of Sciences, and most health professionals urge people to reduce their salt intake.

As to the other techniques — the jury is still out regarding the effectiveness of voluntary relaxation on long-term blood pressure control. Calcium supplementation with people who are calcium-deficient and hypertensive reduces the blood pressure of some of these candidates. Evidence is beginning to indicate that increasing consumption of potassium-rich foods, particularly from healthy sources such as fruits, vegetables, and whole grains, can prevent or lower blood pressure.[14]

Aerobic exercises, such as walking and jogging, help to control blood pressure. Based on the evidence, the American College of Sports Medicine (ACSM) has taken the position that "endurance (aerobic) exercise training by individuals at high risk for developing hypertension will reduce the rise in blood pressure that occurs with time."[15] Furthermore, aerobic exercises performed at moderate intensity (40% to 70% of aerobic capacity) seem to lower blood pressure as much as, and sometimes more than, exercises performed at higher intensities.

How does aerobic exercise lower blood pressure? *First*, epinephrine and norepinephrine are hormones secreted by the body that play important roles in regulating blood pressure. Both are **vasoconstrictors**; they clamp down on the **arterioles**, which requires more force to circulate blood through them. Aerobic training decreases the circulating levels of these hormones, which allows the arterioles to relax and widen. Exercise keeps the arteries limber. This response lowers the resistance to blood flow, which in turn lowers the blood pressure.

Second, aerobic exercise increases cells' sensitivity to insulin. **Insulin** is a hormone the body manufactures that facilitates the passage of sugar from the blood to the cells. Sugar (glucose) is an important source of energy the cells use to perform their normal functions. Increased sensitivity to insulin yields an important bonus: Excess sodium is excreted by the kidneys, and this also lowers the blood pressure. *Third*, aerobic exercise contributes to weight loss, which lowers the blood pressure.

High Serum Cholesterol

Cholesterol is a steroid required for the manufacture of hormones and bile (for the digestion and absorption of fats); it is one of the structural components of neural tissue; and it is required for the construction of cell walls. Although a certain amount of cholesterol is needed for good health, an excessive amount in the blood — **serum cholesterol** — is associated with heart attacks and strokes. Strokes, or "brain attacks," are a result of blood clots blocking the flow of blood to portions of the brain or a hemorrhage in the brain resulting from a blood vessel that has burst (see Figure 5.3). Common consequences of a stroke are paralysis of one side of the body and slurred speech. If a stroke is massive, the victim dies.

Humans obtain cholesterol in two ways

1. External, through dietary consumption
2. Internal, by the body manufacturing its own.

The average male consumes 376 milligrams (mg) of cholesterol daily, and females, 259 milligrams a day.[16] The American Heart Association (AHA) recommends daily consumption of less than 300 mg. This is compared to a dietary intake of cholesterol by males in 1960 of 706 mg per day, while females were consuming 493 mg per day. We have made significant progress in reducing our dietary cholesterol over the last three decades. But, we need no dietary intake of cholesterol because the liver manufactures all of the cholesterol the body needs.

Saturated fat is the primary ingredient from which cholesterol is produced inside the body. As a result, most authorities are more concerned about the amount of saturated fat, rather than cholesterol we consume, but they are quick to add that it is prudent to limit the intake of both.

Dietary cholesterol and saturated fat are found in animal flesh, eggs, whole milk, and whole-milk dairy products. Fruits and vegetables are free of cholesterol, and — with a few exceptions — are also low in fat. Coconuts, coconut oil, palm oil, and palm kernel oil are high in saturated fat. Olives, nuts and seeds, and avocados are high in monounsaturated fat, which is a less harmful form. Regardless, AHA guidelines indicate that consumption of fat should be less than 30% of the total caloric intake.

The amount of cholesterol circulating in the blood is expressed in milligrams per deciliter (mg/dL), so a cholesterol level of 210 is read as 210 mg/dL. Table 5.3 indicates levels of risk for serum cholesterol.

Maintaining a desirable value of serum cholesterol reduces the risk. For every 1% that serum cholesterol is lowered, the risk of heart disease is reduced by 2% to 3%.[17]

Cholesterol Carriers   Knowing one's total serum cholesterol value tells only part of the story. To fully evaluate the cholesterol risk, we must know our total cholesterol (TC) as well as two of its important fractions — the low density lipoprotein (LDL) fraction and the high density lipoprotein (HDL) fraction. The **lipoproteins** are carriers to which cholesterol attaches for transport through the circulatory system.

The most atherogenic (capable of producing atherosclerosis) of the carriers is the **LDL** group. This fraction is the primary transporter of cholesterol from the liver to the cells of the body. The liver and cells have receptor sites that lock onto the LDLs so their cargo of cholesterol and other fats can be assimilated for use by them. Under normal conditions, the cells effectively

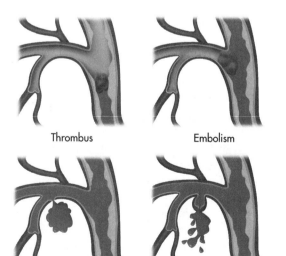

Thrombus   Embolism

Hemorrhage   Aneurysm

Figure 5.3   Causes of stroke.

Table 5.3 Relative Risks of Serum Cholesterol

Cholesterol (mg/dL)	Level of Risk
< 200*	Desirable
200–239	Borderline
≥ 240**	High

* < less than
** ≥ equal to or greater than

remove cholesterol from circulation, but when LDL concentrations are excessive, the receptor sites become saturated, impeding further removal. The net result is a rise in blood concentrations of both LDL and cholesterol.

Excess LDLs are oxidized in the cells of the artery walls. This is the beginning of atherosclerosis and the formation of plaques that eventually clog the arteries that supply blood to the heart and brain. The LDL concentration may be lowered through weight loss and reduction in the intake of saturated fat, total fat, and cholesterol. Table 5.4 presents the relative risk associated with LDL cholesterol.

A second important cholesterol carrier is the high density lipoprotein (HDL) fraction. The **HDLs** are involved in reverse transport; they scavenge cholesterol from the tissues and bloodstream and transfer it back to the liver through intermediary carriers, for degradation, recycling, or disposal. HDLs protect the arteries from atherosclerosis by clearing cholesterol from the blood. The higher the HDL count, the better. A low number of circulating HDLs is a powerful independent predictor of heart disease. Table 5.5 presents HDL values and their relative risk.

HDLs can be increased through aerobic exercise, weight loss, and moderate alcohol intake. "Moderate intake" means approximately one ounce of alcohol per day for males and 1/2 ounce for females. Approximately one-half to two-thirds of an ounce is found in 12 ounces of beer, 5 ounces of wine, and 1.5 ounces of 80-proof spirits. Alcohol also can be a substance of abuse, and overuse or misuse contributes to 100,000 deaths annually in the United States.[18]

Be careful regarding your alcohol intake. It has a lot of calories, second only to fat. Avoid alcohol if you are watching your weight, if you intend to drive, or if anyone in your family has alcoholic tendencies.

Table 5.5 HDL Values and Degree of Relative Risk by Gender

HDL Cholesterol (mg/dL)	Risk
45	Average for males
55	Average for females
< 25	Triple the risk for males
< 40*	Triple the risk for females

* < less than

Determining Cholesterol Risk An accurate assessment of the cholesterol risk requires measurement of total cholesterol (TC) and the LDL and HDL fractions. A desirable total cholesterol still can put one at significant risk if the LDLs are too high or the HDLs are too low. Another clue regarding risk is provided by the ratio between total cholesterol and HDL. Dividing total cholesterol by HDL yields an index number that is interpreted with the aid of Table 5.6.

Physical Inactivity

Physical inactivity is debilitating to the human body. Humans are exponents of the biological dictate "use it or lose it." That which we use becomes stronger, while that which we do not use becomes weaker. All body systems and all muscles, including the heart muscle, respond to this principle.

The results of a number of important investigations have concluded that physical inactivity is major risk for heart disease. Those who exercise consistently, even at low intensity, tend to be

Table 5.4 Guidelines for LDL Cholesterol Risk

LDL Cholesterol (mg/dL)	Risk
< 130*	Desirable
130–159	Borderline-High
> 160**	High

* < less than
** > greater than

Table 5.6 Ratio of Total Cholesterol to HDL

Risk	Male	Female
Very Low (½ of average)	< 3.4*	< 3.3
Low	4.0	3.8
Average	5.0	4.5
Moderate (2 × average)	9.5	7.0
High (3 × average)	> 23**	> 11.0

* < less than
** > greater than

healthier and to live longer than people who are sedentary. The ongoing Harvard Alumni Study found that the minimum exercise threshold for increasing longevity was as little as walking five miles per week.[19] Those who walked or jogged 20 to 22 miles per week achieved optimal benefits. They lived an average of 2 years longer than sedentary people.

Investigators at the Cooper Institute for Aerobics Research found that physically fit subjects who had high blood pressure or elevated serum cholesterol were less likely to die prematurely from all causes than unfit individuals with normal values of both.[20] The Centers for Disease Control and Prevention concluded that exercise is the one lifestyle change that could most affect health status.[21] This is based primarily on the fact that more than 60% of Americans are either sedentary or exercise too infrequently to enhance their health.

Health enhancement through physical activity does not require a great deal of effort. The requirement is 30 minutes of physical activity at least four days per week every week. There are few constraints on the type of activities that can be chosen. All physical activities (cycling, jogging, walking, swimming, etc), most games and sports, many leisure-time activities, and some occupational work have the potential to meet the minimum criteria for improving health. Exercise, in sum, has the following cardiovascular benefits:

1. Increases HDL-cholesterol
2. Decreases LDL-cholesterol
3. Favorably changes the ratios between total cholesterol and HDL-C, and between LDL-C and HDL-cholesterol
4. Decreases triglyceride levels
5. Promotes relaxation; relieves stress and tension
6. Decreases body fat and favorably changes body composition
7. Reduces blood pressure especially if it is high
8. Blood platelets are less sticky
9. Results in fewer cardiac arrhythmias
10. Increases myocardial efficiency
    a. Lowers resting heart rate
    b. Increases stroke volume
11. Increases oxygen-carrying capacity of the blood

Exercise on a regular basis has been emphasized in this text because it is the *only* way to improve fitness and health simultaneously. Another important reason for consistent participation in exercise is that it reduces the risk of sudden death from a heart attack during and immediately after sporadic physical exertion (such as shoveling snow). Two studies, one completed in the United States and the other in Germany, documented this observation. The U.S. study showed that sedentary people were 100 times more vulnerable to suffering a heart attack during strenuous activity than at other times.[22] In contrast, those who exercise consistently face only a small increase in the risk, but the health and fitness benefits that are achieved from training far outweigh the minimal risk.[23]

Obesity

The current perception of obesity is that it is a chronic disease like hypertension or diabetes rather than a simple failure of willpower.[24] Data indicate that Americans once again are gaining weight. The number of overweight males has risen from 24% to 32%, and the number of overweight females has risen from 27% to 35%.

Excess body weight carries medical consequences. Obesity increases the risk and the consequences of many other chronic diseases. It significantly increases the workload of the heart, and it coexists with high blood pressure and elevated serum cholesterol. Obesity is related to the onset of diabetes, arthritis, and some forms of cancer.

The National Institutes of Health defines **obesity** as 20% above desirable weight. Other authorities define it relative to the percent of body weight that consists of fat. This is a more accurate method that provides guidelines for weight loss and weight control. Males are obese when 25% or more of their total body weight is in the form of fat. Females are obese when 32% or more of their total body weight is in the form of fat.

Excessive fat is a risk, and the manner in which it is distributed also has to be considered. Abdominal fat — also known as android, central, and masculine pattern fat — increases the risk for heart attacks, stroke, diabetes, and some forms of cancer. Even as few as 15 extra pounds stored in this pattern increases the risk substantially. Fat that is stored in the hips, buttocks, and thighs — also known as gynoid fat and feminine pattern fat — presents less of a risk.

Fortunately, obesity is reversible. When the excess weight is lost, the risk subsides. Weight loss strategies are discussed in Chapter 7.

Other Contributing Factors

Diabetes Mellitus

Diabetes mellitus is a metabolic disorder in which the body is unable to regulate the level of blood glucose (sugar). It is one of the 10 leading causes of death in the United States. Diabetics who die prematurely succumb to complications of the disease. These include cardiovascular lesions, accelerated atherosclerosis, and heart disease. Diabetics also are susceptible to kidney disease, nerve and blood vessel damage, blindness, and lower-limb amputation resulting from gangrene. In addition, diabetes tends to elevate serum cholesterol and creates an environment in the circulatory system that facilitates the development of blood clots. Many physicians are

convinced that diabetes is a major risk for coronary heart disease.[25]

The two types of diabetes mellitus are:

1. *Type I* — usually occurring early in life. Victims of Type I diabetes don't produce insulin, so they must take it by daily injection. Insulin is a hormone that regulates blood sugar by moving it, when appropriate, from the blood to the cells, where it can be used to fuel the cell's needs. Without insulin, sugar would accumulate in the blood and spill out of the body through the kidneys. The body would be forced to use fat as its primary fuel, and this produces serious consequences for the diabetic. Although diabetes cannot be cured, it can be controlled. Living a well-regulated life that includes exercise, weight control, and a low-fat diet is paramount to controlling Type I diabetes.

2. *Type II* — occurring about middle age to overweight, underactive people. This form of diabetes may or may not require medication. Lifestyle factors are important in the treatment and control of Type II diabetes. Exercise and weight loss combine to increase cellular sensitivity to insulin so blood sugar can be normalized with less insulin. Each exercise bout reduces blood platelet adhesiveness for about 24 hours. This lessens the advent of a heart attack by decreasing the likelihood of a coronary spasm. Many physicians encourage their diabetic patients to walk as the preferred form of exercise.

A landmark piece of research, The Physician's Health Study, was a large-scale collaborative effort. It showed that exercise reduced the risk of developing Type II diabetes.[26] Type II accounts for 90% of all cases of diabetes. Physicians who exercised vigorously five or more times per week had a 42% reduction in the incidence of Type II diabetes compared to those who exercised less than once a week. Each 500 calories burned per week in physical activity reduces the risk of Type II diabetes by 6%.[27] The reduction in the risk was particularly evident in those at greatest risk — the obese. The researchers concluded that at least 24% of all Type II diabetes was related to a sedentary lifestyle.

Stress

Although stress is difficult to quantify, authorities tend to agree that chronic stress or distress produces physiological changes in the body that can predispose people to illness. Stress also hastens the process of **subclinical disease.**

Chronic stress can have a detrimental effect on the immune system for months or years. Stress stimulates the secretion of above normal amounts of hormones, collectively called the **catecholamines**, that circulate at high levels in the bloodstream. The catecholamines rev up the body's engine so it runs at high throttle. Physical exercise is the antidote because it metabolizes these products and thereby lowers their level in the blood. But the catecholamine level of sedentary people remains elevated so the arterioles are in a constant state of slight contraction. This condition, known as **peripheral vascular resistance**, increases the workload of the heart. Aerobic exercise reduces peripheral vascular resistance, decreases the severity of the stress response, shortens the recovery time from stress, and reduces stress-related vulnerability to disease.

Situations and circumstances are stressful only if we allow them to be. The stressor is not what produces the problem. It is the way we perceive and react to it. Two people confronted by the same stressor might exhibit different reactions. For example, delivering a speech to a group of people is anxiety-producing and threatening to one of them and is an exciting challenge to another. We cannot avoid stress. It is part of life in our competitive, dynamic society.

We currently are entering the age of information. This will provide rapid changes in our educational and occupational lives. The information superhighway will compound the normal stressful life-change events that occur to many of us.

Divorce, death of a loved one, layoff from a job, and retirement are among the stressful events we might have to deal with. Because we cannot avoid stress, we must learn to manage it. Exercise is a beneficial coping mechanism that rids the body of stress-initiated harmful products that accumulate over time.

New and Emerging Risk Factors

Research has increased our knowledge of risk factors for cardiovascular disease. Two advances relate to homocysteine and another form of lipoprotein.

Homocysteine

Homocysteine is one of the amino-acid building blocks of protein. It is carried in the blood, and under normal conditions it splits into two other amino acids. When it does not split, homocysteine blood levels rise, increasing the risk for heart disease. Several major studies have shown that the probability of having a heart attack rises to three times above normal in people who have the highest homocysteine levels. This puts this risk factor on a par with the other major risk factors for coronary heart disease.[28]

High homocysteine levels damage the inner lining of the arteries. The lesions, or injuries, that it causes stimulate the abnormal growth of smooth muscle cells in the artery walls, which in turn promote the development and progression of atherosclerosis. Homocysteine levels can be controlled through proper diet. The B vitamins folic acid (folate), B_6, and B_{12} are needed to process homocysteine. Of the three, **folic acid** is the most important, but maximum results are attained when all three are available to the body in optimal amounts. The recommended daily intake is 400 micrograms (mcg) of folate, 6 micrograms of B_{12}, and 2 milligrams (mg) of B_6.

Lipoprotein (a)

Lipoprotein (a) represents a group of particles that resemble low density lipoprotein (LDL-C), which is the most harmful form of cholesterol. Many scientists believe that high levels of **Lp(a)** promote the development of blood clots in the arteries. In addition, they enhance the plaque-forming ability of LDL-C.

Plaque is the material that grows inside the walls of arteries, narrowing the diameter of these vessels. Lp(a) may be as dangerous to the heart and its blood vessels as low levels of HDL-C (the protective form of cholesterol).[29]

Lp(a) levels are determined primarily by genetic make-up. Therefore, people with high blood levels should concentrate on lowering risk factors over which they have control such as total cholesterol and its sub-fractions, blood pressure, body weight, and tobacco usage. Equally important is a regular exercise program.

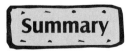

Summary

- The leading form of cardiovascular disease, claiming about half a million lives annually, is coronary heart disease.

- Coronary heart disease is characterized by obstructions (blood clots or spasms) in the coronary arteries that lead to a reduction or stoppage of blood flow to portions of the heart muscle.

- Atherosclerosis is a slow, progressive disease of large and mid-size arteries.

- Risk factors are genetic or learned behaviors that increase the probability of premature illness and death from a specific chronic disease.

- The statistical probability that death will occur from heart disease increases with advancing age.

- Children whose parents have heart disease or atherosclerosis have an increased tendency to develop these conditions.

- Cigarette smoking is responsible for nearly a third of mortality from heart disease.

- Smoking is rising among teenagers of both sexes.

- Nicotine is a powerful addictive stimulant that has profound adverse effect on the cardiovascular system.

- The carbon monoxide in cigarette smoke displaces oxygen and reduces the oxygen-carrying capacity of the blood.

- The danger of cigarette smoking is measured in pack-years.

- Breathing secondhand smoke is harmful to nonsmokers.

- Smokeless tobacco products are addictive and harmful.

- Essential hypertension is the most common form of high blood pressure.

- Lifestyle behaviors that can prevent or treat hypertension include exercise, weight loss, salt restriction, optimum calcium and potassium intake, and voluntary relaxation techniques.

- Cholesterol is found in animal flesh, eggs, whole milk, and whole-milk dairy products. Its consumption in the United States has been decreasing since 1960.

- The liver manufactures cholesterol from saturated fat, the human body does not have to supply it; therefore, our intake of this form of fat should be minimal.

- LDL cholesterol is implicated in the development of atherosclerosis.

- HDL cholesterol protects the arteries by removing cholesterol from the blood.

- People who exercise consistently tend to be healthier and live longer than people who are sedentary.

- The risk of sudden death during and immediately after exercise is much more likely in unfit people.

- The number of overweight people has increased notably.

- Obesity is considered a disease and is a risk factor for other chronic diseases as well.

- The android pattern of fat deposition increases the risk of heart disease, stroke, diabetes, and some forms of cancer.

- Diabetes mellitus is a metabolic disorder in which the body is unable to regulate the level of blood glucose.

- Type I diabetes usually appears early in life and requires the daily injection of insulin.

- Type II diabetes usually arises about middle-age to overweight and underexercised people. The Physician's Health Study concluded that a least 24% of all Type II diabetes is related to a sedentary lifestyle.

- Stress suppresses the immune system. Because we cannot avoid stress, we must learn to manage it.

- Homocysteine in the blood damages the arteries and increases the risk for heart attack.

- Lp(a) increases the likelihood of developing blood clots and forming plaque in the arteries.

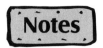

Notes

1. D. L. Hoyert, K. D. Kochanek, and S. L. Murphy, "Deaths: Final Data for 1997," *National Vital Statistics Reports*, 47:19 (June 30, 1999).
2. AHA.
3. AHA.
4. S. Grundy, "Decline in Coronary Heart Disease Mortality: Primary Factors and Secondary Interventions," *Cholesterol and Coronary Disease — Reducing the Risk*, 4:4 (1993), 1.
5. "Old Habits: Will You Pay For Your Past as a Smoker?" *Harvard Health Letter*, 23:8 (June 1998), 1–3.
6. U. S. Department of Health and Human Services, *Physical Activity and Health: A Report of the Surgeon General* (Atlanta: U. S. Dept. of Health and Human Services, Centers for Disease Control and Prevention, National Center for Chronic Disease Prevention and Health Promotion, 1996).
7. Grundy.
8. U. S. Dept. of Health, Surgeon General's Report, 1996.
9. Harvard Health Letter.
10. American Cancer Society, *Cancer Facts and Figures — 1997* (Atlanta: American Cancer Society, 1997).
11. Smoking Cessation Clinical Practice Guidelines Panel and Staff, "The Agency for Health Care Policy and Research Smoking Cessation Clinical Practice Guidelines," *Journal of the American Medical Association*, 275 (1996), 1270–1280.

12. D. J. Anspaugh, M. H. Hamrick, and F. D. Rosato, *Wellness Concepts and Applications* (St. Louis: McGraw-Hill, 1997).
13. B. Liebman, "The Salt Shake-out," *Nutrition Action Health Letter*, 21:2 (March 1994), 5.
14. "High Blood Pressure Lifestyle Changes Replace Drugs for Some," *Harvard Health Letter*, 23:7 (May 1998), 5.
15. American College of Sports Medicine, "Physical Activity, Physical Fitness, and Hypertension," *Medicine and Science in Sports and Exercise*, 25:10 (1993), i.
16. "Fascinating Facts," *University of California at Berkeley Wellness Letter*, 10:6 (March 1994), 1.
17. J. C. La Rosa et al., "The Cholesterol Facts: A Summary of the Evidence Relating Dietary Fats, Serum Cholesterol, and Coronary Heart Disease: A Joint Statement by the American Heart Association and the National Heart Lung, and Blood Institute," *Circulation*, 81 (1990), 1721.
18. J. D. Potter and F. Hutchinson, "Hazards and Benefits of Alcohol," *New England Journal of Medicine*, 337:24 (Dec. 11, 1997), 1763–1764.
19. I-M Lee, C. Hsieh, and R. S. Paffenbarger, "Exercise Intensity and Longevity in Men: The Harvard Alumni Health Study," *Journal of the American Medical Association*, 273:5 (April 19, 1995), 1179–1184.

20. S. N. Blair et al., "Changes in Physical Fitness and All-Cause Mortality," *Journal of the American Medical Association*, 273:14 (April 12, 1995), 1093–1098.
21. K. E. Powell et al., "Physical Activity and the Incidence of Coronary Heart Disease," *Annual Review of Public Health*, 8 (1987), 253.
22. M. A. Mittleman et al., "Triggering of Acute Myocardial Infarction By Heavy Physical Exertion," *New England Journal of Medicine*, 329 (1993), 1677.
23. S. N. Willich et al., "Physical Exertion as a Trigger of Acute Myocardial Infarction," *New England Journal of Medicine*, 329 (1993), 1684.
24. U. S. Dept. of Health and Human Services, Report of the Surgeon General, 1996.
25. AHA.
26. J. E. Manson et al., "A Prospective Study of Exercise and Incidence of Diabetes Among U. S. Male Physicians," *Journal of the American Medical Association*, 268 (1992), 268.
27. U. S. Dept. of Health and Human Services, Report of the Surgeon General, 1996.
28. "Evidence Mounts for Heart Disease Marker," *Harvard Health Letter*, 22:11 (Sept. 1997), 1–3.
29. "Ask the Experts," *U. C. Berkeley Wellness Letter*, 14:3 (Dec. 1997), 7.

Reducing the Risk for Chronic Diseases

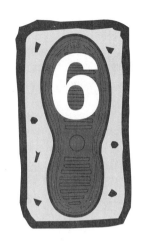

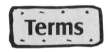

Allergen

Asthmogenic

Carcinogenic

Clinical depression

Distress

Eustress

Malignant

Metastasis

Neoplasm

Oncogene

Peristalsis

Stressors

Hormone replacement
    therapy (HRT

This chapter focuses on the chronic diseases of cancer, osteoporosis, osteoarthritis, and asthma, as well as stress. These conditions were selected because of their prevalence in the United States and because they are related to exercise. Exercising regularly has a modifying or preventive effect on each of these diseases and can mitigate against stress, which is a contributor to many of the chronic diseases.

CANCER

Cancer, the second leading cause of death in the U.S., is responsible for one in every five deaths.[1] Projected estimates for 1999 indicated that 563,100 people would die from cancer and 1,221,800 new cases would be diagnosed. The incidence of cancer has been on the increase during the last 60 years. A large part of the rise consists of lung cancer in both men and women. If lung cancer deaths were excluded, total mortality from cancer would have declined by 16% during this period. Figure 6.1 shows the deaths from lung cancer in the United States.

Cancer is actually a general term that applies to more than 100 diseases characterized by abnormal and uncontrolled cellular growth. Any cell can become cancerous if it is exposed under the right conditions to **carcinogenic** (cancer-producing) substances. Exposure to carcinogens eventually will give rise to mutant cells, which will divide and grow uncontrollably. Normal cells follow an orderly and predictable blueprint for growth and division. In adulthood this is restricted to the replacement of lost cells. Cancerous cells do not respond to the body's signals restricting cellular division, so they and their offspring continue to grow wildly. The mass of new growth is a tumor or **neoplasm** (new tissue).

Cancerous tumors are **malignant**. They grow rapidly, and they are not confined or localized. They shed their cells, invade surrounding tissues, and compete with normal cells for space and nutrients. **Metastasis** is the medical term for the spread of cancer from its original site to other areas of the body. The processes that transform normal cells to malignant ones are complex and not well understood. Normal genes that undergo mutation may become **oncogenes**, or cancerous genes. When oncogenes divide, they pass on their malignant characteristics to their progeny. Scientists are attempting to identify the products manufactured and given off by oncogenes. If these are distinguishable, they can be used as markers to detect cancer in its earliest and most treatable stage.

Techniques and strategies have emerged that can reduce the incidence of many forms of cancer. Cancer prevention includes:

- abstinence from all forms of tobacco
- a diet rich in fruits, vegetables, and grains, is low in fat, and devoid of smoked and cured meat and fish
- minimum exposure to radiation and carcinogenic chemicals
- regular participation in exercise.

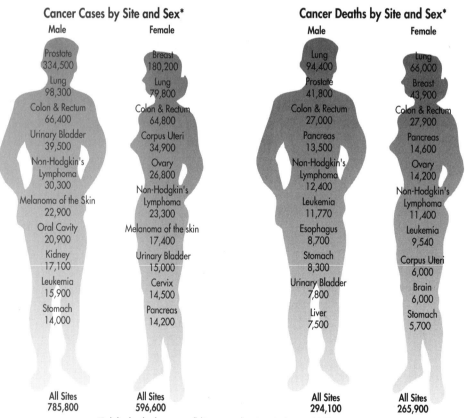

Cancer Cases by Site and Sex*

Male	Female
Prostate 334,500	Breast 180,200
Lung 98,300	Lung 79,800
Colon & Rectum 66,400	Colon & Rectum 64,800
Urinary Bladder 39,500	Corpus Uteri 34,900
Non-Hodgkin's Lymphoma 30,300	Ovary 26,800
Melanoma of the Skin 22,900	Non-Hodgkin's Lymphoma 23,300
Oral Cavity 20,900	Melanoma of the skin 17,400
Kidney 17,100	Urinary Bladder 15,000
Leukemia 15,900	Cervix 14,500
Stomach 14,000	Pancreas 14,200
All Sites 785,800	All Sites 596,600

Cancer Deaths by Site and Sex*

Male	Female
Lung 94,400	Lung 66,000
Prostate 41,800	Breast 43,900
Colon & Rectum 27,000	Colon & Rectum 27,900
Pancreas 13,500	Pancreas 14,600
Non-Hodgkin's Lymphoma 12,400	Ovary 14,200
Leukemia 11,770	Non-Hodgkin's Lymphoma 11,400
Esophagus 8,700	Leukemia 9,540
Stomach 8,300	Corpus Uteri 6,000
Urinary Bladder 7,800	Brain 6,000
Liver 7,500	Stomach 5,700
All Sites 294,100	All Sites 265,900

*Excluding basal and squamous cell skin cancer and carcinoma in situ except bladder.

Figure 6.1 1998 cancer incidence and deaths by site and sex.

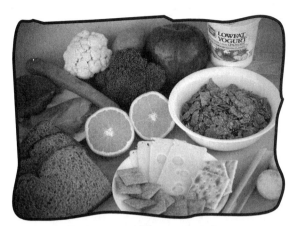

Fruits, vegetables, and grains:
a healthy anti-cancer diet.

Exercise diminishes the risk of colon cancer and possibly breast cancer, and might slow the progression of other malignancies as well.[2] Mortality from all types of cancer was highest in those who were the least physically active, compared to those who were the most physically active, in the Harvard Alumni Study.[3] At the Cooper Institute for Aerobics Research, the most physically fit of 13,344 subjects had the lowest incidence of all forms of cancer, while the least fit had the highest.[4]

A number of investigations have examined the relationship between physical activity and site-specific cancers. Conclusions from more than two dozen studies indicate that regular exercise reduces the risk of colon cancer, the third leading cause of death by cancer for males and females.[5]

Regular exercise protects the colon by stimulating colonic **peristalsis,** the waves of alternate contraction and relaxation that propel digested food along the colon. This action shortens the transit time of the fecal stream through this vessel. Heightened peristaltic action reduces contact between potential carcinogens in fecal matter and the walls of the colon.

Studies that have investigated the relationship between physical exercise and breast cancer have produced mixed results. Moderate or vigorous exercise performed regularly might protect against breast cancer by reducing the output of estrogen, a known causative factor in the development of this disease. Second, regular exercise promotes loss of fat and weight. A number of studies have indicated that the leanest subjects had the lowest production of estrogen and the lowest incidence of breast cancer.[6] Breast cancer is the second leading cause of cancer deaths in women.[7]

Several studies investigating the relationship between physical exercise and prostate cancer found no consistent result.[8] Nevertheless, the biological plausibility of a protective relationship exists. Prostate cancer is related to the production of testosterone, the male sex hormone, and vigorous physical exercise decreases the manufacture of this product to some extent. Therefore, reduced circulating levels of testosterone might result in lowered risk for prostate cancer, which is the second leading cause of death from cancer among men.[9]

Exercise possibly plays another role in preventing and combating cancer: It stimulates the immune system to increase the production of cancer-fighting chemicals and improves the cancer-killing power of certain cells. Moderate amounts of exercise at moderate intensity seem

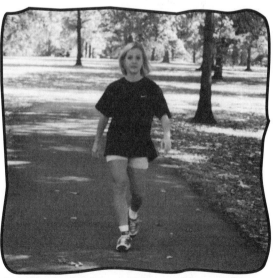

Regular moderate exercises — such as walking —
strengthen the immune system.

to promote these functions best, whereas prolonged, vigorous exercise could depress the effectiveness of the immune system. Highly trained endurance-type competitive athletes often report an increase in the common cold, flu, and upper respiratory infections during heavy training and after competition. This is an indicator of a weakened immune system.[10] Even though very heavy exercise might depress the immune system, the problem for most people in the United States is too little exercise rather than too much.

OSTEOPOROSIS

Osteoporosis literally means "porous bone." It is a "silent condition" characterized by the gradual loss of bone mass. As a result, the bones become brittle and vulnerable to fracturing as we age. Two types of osteoporosis have been identified: primary and secondary. Primary osteoporosis, the most prevalent form, is the result of normal physiological processes that include aging and menopause.[11] Type I primary osteoporosis refers to accelerated bone loss that accompanies the declining level of estrogen during and after menopause. Bone loss declines rapidly for 3 to 7 years after menopause, and then plateaus. Type II primary osteoporosis is age-related and is characterized by a gradual loss of bone. It usually is not apparent until 75 years of age or so. This form of osteoporosis affects both men and women.

Secondary osteoporosis arises from some identifiable medical condition such as diabetes, liver disease, and rheumatoid arthritis, among others. Medications also might contribute to the development of secondary osteoporosis.

The most common fracture sites associated with osteoporosis are vertebral crush fractures (bones of the spinal column) and fractures of the hip, wrist, and femur (thigh bone). The annual cost of this devastating disease is estimated to exceed $60 billion by the year 2000. In addition to this economic burden, the death rate within the first year after a hip fracture in an elderly person is 18% to 33%, and most of those who survive have a diminished quality of life.[12]

Risk Factors for Osteoporosis

Some factors that increase the likelihood of developing osteoporosis are outlined as follows.

♦ *Age:* Osteoporosis takes many years to develop, so the longer a person lives, the greater is the probability of his or her developing this disease.

♦ *Gender:* Women are more susceptible than men, particularly those with a small, thin skeletal framework and those who experience early menopause. **Hormone replacement therapy (HRT)** during and after menopause might be necessary. The decision to take HRT should be based on risk versus benefit, and it should be made by patient and physician together.

♦ *Heredity:* The offspring of parents who have osteoporosis are at greater risk.

♦ *Lack of physical activity:* Weight-bearing exercises and resistance exercises increase the strength and thickness of bones. Conversely, lack of stimulation from sedentary living contributes to the loss of bone minerals.

♦ *Cigarette smoking:* Cigarette smoking suppresses estrogen levels and leads to premature menopause so bone loss occurs earlier in life.

♦ *Insufficient intake of calcium and vitamin D:* The National Institutes of Health (NIH) recommends that premenopausal women should take at least 1000 milligrams (mg) of calcium daily. Postmenopausal women under 65 years of age who are taking estrogen replacement also should take at least 1000 mg. Postmenopausal women who are not taking estrogen need 1500 mg of calcium, and all men and women older than 65 years of age also need 1500 mg.

Vitamin D is necessary to aid in the absorption of calcium from the intestines. The daily intake that is recommended for this purpose is 400 to 800 international units (IU).

Osteoporosis is treatable, but it is not curable. The best approach is to prevent or delay its advent. The most important preventive technique is to develop as much bone as possible during the teenage years. Peak bone density occurs between ages of 20 and 30, but 90% of adult bone mineral content is deposited by the end of adolescence.[13] To achieve this increase involves a sufficient intake of calcium and vitamin D, and a regular program of weight-bearing and resistance-type exercise. Unfortunately, most female teenagers do neither, thereby setting themselves up for skeletal problems later in life.

Effects of Exercise

Bone is living tissue that responds to the downward force of gravity and the lateral forces generated by the forceful contraction of muscles. Weight-bearing, impact-loading exercises such as walking, jogging, aerobic dancing, and stair climbing can increase bone mass.[14] Even the

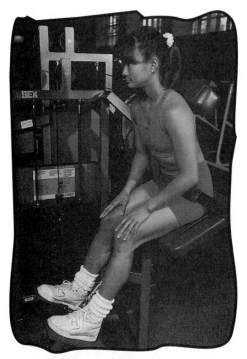

Resistance exercises protect
the skeletal system from osteoporosis.

skeletal systems of nursing-home residents (average age 87 years) have responded to exercise with an increase in bone mass. Nonweight-bearing activities such as swimming and stationary cycling are not as effective in increasing bone density.[15]

Researchers have examined the effect of resistance weight training on the skeletal system. Studies have indicated that bones respond to weight training by becoming thicker and denser.[16] For good results, weight-training exercises should be done at an intensity level equal to 80% of 1 repetition maximum (1RM). This is approximately equivalent to performing 10 lifts, or repetitions, of an exercise with a weight heavy enough so it cannot be lifted 11 times. Exercises that stress the major muscle groups should be selected so the bones to which they are attached also will be stressed.

OSTEOARTHRITIS

Osteoarthritis is the most common of the many forms of arthritis. Osteoarthritis leads to decline of the soft, smooth cartilage at the surface of joints. This happens to some people as early as 30 years of age.

The two types of osteoarthritis are primary and secondary. Primary osteoarthritis is the result of normal use and is referred to as "wear-and-tear" arthritis. The joints most commonly affected are the thumb and end joints of the other fingers, the hips, knees, neck, and lower spine.[17] Secondary osteoarthritis can result from one or a combination of the following: (1) joint injury, (2) disease, and, (3) chronic traumas imposed by obesity, poor posture, and occupational overuse. Osteoarthritis causes minimal inflammation of the affected joints.

One of the myths that seems to persist is that jogging causes premature osteoarthritis of the knees. This perception is fueled by the biomechanics of jogging which indicates that the force developed at the knee when the foot strikes the ground is six times that of the force generated by walking. As a result, many have concluded that jogging must be harmful to the knees. However, 35 years of data collected by researchers in the Framingham Heart Study indicated that the major cause of osteoarthritis of the knees is obesity.[18] In fact, high mileage running — an average of 28 miles per week for a minimum of 12 years — was not associated with the premature development of osteoarthritis. A later study confirmed the Framingham conclusion. This investigation found that persons in the upper 20% of body weight experienced 7 to 10 times the risk of developing osteoarthritis of the knees and hips than those whose body weight was in the lowest 20%.[19]

Osteoarthritics need to exercise because it increases strength, promotes flexibility, reduces pain, controls body weight, preserves mobility, and enhances well-being.[20] The health of cartilage, which has no blood supply of its own, depends on regular stimulation and use of the joints. When the joints move, fluid and waste products are squeezed out of cartilage. When the joint relaxes, fluid seeps back in, bringing oxygen and nutrients with it. Rhythmic contractions of the muscles lubricate and nourish the joints.

If osteoarthritis is present already, impact loading exercises could aggravate the condition and produce pain. If this occurs, a simple shift to low-impact nonweight-bearing exercises should bring relief and allow continued participation. Appropriate activities include walking, water walking, water aerobics, and swimming. Other acceptable activities include the use of stationary cycles, rowing machines, and cross-country ski machines.

ASTHMA

The American Thoracic Society defines asthma as the increased responsiveness of the trachea (windpipe) and bronchi (the two main subdivisions of the trachea that transport air to and from the lungs) to a variety of stimuli resulting in airway obstruction that is reversible spontaneously or as a result of treatment. Breathing becomes difficult during an asthma attack, and this can be frightening.

In the United States, 14 million people are asthmatic and more than 5,000 die from asthma-related conditions each year.[21] Asthma affects about 5% of all Americans.[22] Although asthma has no cure, medications are available to effectively prevent or reduce the length and severity of an attack.

Many potential triggering mechanisms, or **allergens**, can provoke an asthma attack. These include cold, dry air, exercise, viral infections, emotions, sinus infection, and environmental irritants, among others.

Although asthmatics often remain sedentary because of their fear of exercise-induced asthma (EIA), asthma should not be a deterrent to children, adolescents, and older adults participating in physical activities. The American Academy of Allergy and Immunology encourages regular exercise for asthmatics, who receive the same health benefits as other individuals. People with asthma have competed in sports at the national and international levels. In 1984, 11% of the U.S. Olympic Team consisted of athletes who had asthma or exercise-induced asthma.[23] Collectively, these asthmatic athletes — 67 of them — won 41 Olympic medals. Their successful participation was possible because of the combination of medical preventive treatment and their high level of physical fitness.

Asthmatics who want to exercise or who currently are exercising can use the same method of prevention that Olympic athletes practiced.

1. Airway-opening drugs should be used immediately prior to exercise or competition.

2. A gradual warm-up period of 15 minutes should be followed by a 15-minute period of rest. This protocol reduces the probability of incurring exercise-induced asthma for about 2 hours.

3. Treatment must be individualized to find the optimal regimen for each individual. This will involve several trial-and-error attempts before determining the best approach.

The types and intensity of exercise that contribute to the onset of exercise-induced asthma have been identified. The mechanisms responsible for EIA are the loss of respiratory heat and water because of the high rate of breathing during exercise. The more intense the exercise, the greater is the loss of heat and water. Therefore, the more intense forms of exercise usually are the most asthmogenic (capable of inducing bronchospasms). Swimming and other water activities are the least asthmogenic types of exercise. This is probably attributable primarily to the warm, moist environment in which they are done and, second, because the high breathing rates necessary to initiate bronchospasms are difficult to achieve.[24] Running and cycling seem to be the most **asthmogenic** of the outdoor activities, but the risk can be minimized by following the guidelines below.[25]

- Take medications as prescribed by your physician.

- Perform a 5- to 10-minute warm-up that includes moderate stretching.

- Gradually increase the pace during the first 10 to 15 minutes of exercise, being careful to keep the heart rate below 140 beats per minute.

- As your physical tolerance to exercise increases, gradually increase the intensity or duration of exercise, or both.

- Breathe slowly through your nose as much as possible because nasal breathing reduces the likelihood of hyperventilation and humidifies and warms the air before it enters the lungs.

- If you exercise outdoors during the winter, breathe through a scarf or mask.

- Avoid exposure to allergens and air pollutants by exercising indoors during air-pollution alerts. Exercise in areas with low auto traffic (for example, public parks, golf courses).

- Recognize that the pollen count is highest in the early morning hours.

- Do a gradual cool-down to avoid rapid thermal changes in the airways.

STRESS

Stress is the nonspecific response of the human organism to any demand, positive or negative, that it encounters. Stress results from any event, condition, or situation that creates change, threat, or loss. These events are referred to as "stress triggers" or simply **stressors**. The effect of potentially stress-producing events, conditions, and circumstances on a given individual depends on the individual's response. When stressors seem to overload or exceed one's ability to cope, the results can be harmful, and the consequences are proportional to the response.

The reaction to a stressor determines its power to induce stress. For example, having to make a speech to a group of people might be a stressor of crisis proportions for one person, whereas the same event might be an exciting challenge to another. We cannot avoid stress. Even if we were to move to a remote mountain hideaway or an uninhabited island, we still could not avoid stress because this type of existence would have its own set of stressful circumstances. Because stress cannot be avoided, the healthy alternative is to learn to manage it. If we apply the short verse attributed to St. Francis of Assissi life's tribulations will be placed in proper context and therefore easier to manage. It states:

> Give me the serenity to accept things I cannot change, courage to change the things I can, and wisdom to know the difference.

The earlier we begin to behave in accordance with this principle, the more gracefully we will be able to cope with the stressful changes in our lives.

Life Events Scale

Researchers indicate that too many changes, bad or good, occurring within a one-year period of time increases the probability of a health-related problem soon after. Figure 6.2 presents the Life Events Scale — Student Version, reflecting the potential effects of 31 stressors, from those requiring the greatest personal adjustment to those requiring the least. Significantly stressful events include death of a loved one, parent's divorce, and being fired from a job. Positive life changes, such as marriage and pregnancy, also are stress-inducing. The former are negative stressors, producing **distress**, and the latter are positive stressors, producing **eustress**. In any case, though, the predictability of life events is limited.

Respond to the changes in your life by checking the items on Figure 6.2 that you have experienced during the past year. Total the points and interpret the results as follows:

1. 300 points or more: high risk of developing a health problem or experiencing a negative health change in the upcoming year.

2. 150–300 points — a 50–50 chance of experiencing a negative health change within 2 years.

3. Under 150 points — a one-in-three chance of experiencing a negative health change in the next couple of years.

Note: Your reaction to life changes, rather than the change itself, is what determines the seriousness of the stress. Deal with life changes constructively by doing the following.

1. Consider what the change means to you personally.

2. Consider the meaning of the change in your life, and focus on your feelings about it.

3. Examine and explore alternatives for adjusting to the change.

4. Think it through before acting. A measured response is usually better than an impulsive one.

5. Pace yourself. Frenetic activity leads to ineffectiveness, and it is a drain on the body's energy reserve.

6. Engage in relaxation activities such as exercise, voluntary relaxation techniques, or other enjoyable activities such as movies, concerts, picnics, or other outings.

7. Follow a regular daily routine as closely as possible.

Event	Life Change Unit
1. Death of a close family member	100
2. Death of a close friend	73
3. Parents' divorce	65
4. Jail term	63
5. Major personal injury or illness	63
6. Marriage	58
7. Fired from job	50
8. Failed important course	47
9. Change in health of family member	45
10. Pregnancy	45
11. Sex problems	44
12. Serious argument with a close friend	40
13. Change in financial status	39
14. Trouble with parents	39
15. Change in major	39
16. New girlfriend or boyfriend	38
17. Increased workload at school	37
18. Outstanding personal achievement	36
19. First quarter/semester in college	35
20. Change in living conditions	31
21. Serious argument with an instructor	30
22. Lower grades than expected	29
23. Change in sleeping habits	29
24. Change in social activities	29
25. Change in eating habits	28
26. Chronic car trouble	26
27. Change in number of family get togethers	26
28. Too many missed classes	25
29. Change of college/change of work	24
30. Dropped more than one class	23
31. Minor traffic violations	20
Your Score	_____
How do you interpret your score?	_____

Health and Wellness, by G. Edlin and E. Golanty (Boston: Jones and Bartlett Publishers, 1992). Reprinted by permission.

Figure 6.2 Life events scale — student version.

8. Talk to family and friends who can be a source of support, as well as objective observers who may be able to offer alternative solutions.

Responses to Stress

Stress can be acute or chronic. *Acute stress* is situational and of short duration. It is the type of stress associated with taking exams, interviewing for a job or changing jobs, and moving to a new apartment. Physiological responses to events such as these (known as the fight-or-flight mechanism) occur immediately before as well as during the event. These include an increase in the secretion of epinephrine, which

— accelerates resting heart rate and blood pressure

— increases the blood supply to the muscles

— decreases blood supply to the digestive system and kidneys

— dilates the pupils of the eyes to take in more information

— increases blood sugar level

— slightly depresses the immune system.

The stressor loses its effect when the event is over, allowing these physiological responses to return to normal. With *chronic stress*, the responses and changes represent a significant strain on the body over time. Examples of chronic stress are having to make quotas and deadlines, working in a job where the employee feels a loss of control, and environments in which one's input is not valued. If people cannot physically or psychologically adapt or separate themselves from the stressor, the ability to resist weakens. Months or years of interacting with a stressor depletes the body's adaptive ability. At some point, the immune system might be compromised, inviting a number of diseases.

Controlling Stress Through Exercise

Several techniques and methods are available for controlling stress. Here we will concentrate specifically on the contribution of exercise. Many studies have indicated that physically fit people subjected to laboratory-induced psychosocial stress exhibit a reduced response to those stressors when compared to unfit people. In addition, they recover from stress more rapidly and are less vulnerable to stress. Several explanations might account for the lower vulnerability to disease and greater sense of well-being:

1. The more robust immune system can ward off infectious diseases and is more efficient in recognizing and destroying mutant cells.

2. In the pyrogenic effect of exercise, the higher body temperature during and immediately after exercise temporarily simulates the fever the body produces naturally in response to viral and bacterial infections. This represents one of the body's defense mechanisms for counteracting disease.

3. Exercise increases the production of endogenous opiates (primarily the beta endorphins) that elevate mood, relieve pain, and provide feelings of relaxation.

4. Exercise lowers blood levels of the catecholamines (epinephrine and norepinephrine) that raise blood pressure by increasing peripheral vascular resistance.

Exercise is beneficial for both body and mind by producing positive physiological and

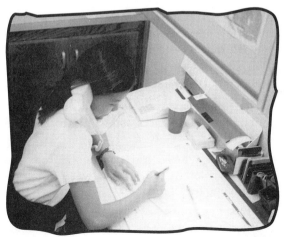

Many people encounter stress daily on the job.

mood changes. People who lose fat and gain muscle become more satisfied with their physical appearance and, as a result, get a lift in self-esteem.

Exercise is an eustressor. It reduces stress and is an outlet for the release of pent-up energy.

DEPRESSION

Clinical depression is prolonged sadness that persists for some time. Symptoms include social withdrawal, feelings of helplessness, and feelings of loss of control over one's life. Exercise is one component in the spectrum of treatments for depression.[26] Studies have shown that aerobic exercises, primarily walking and jogging, have improved the mental health status of depressed patients. Many of these patients improved dramatically enough to be taken off medication, and the improvement of others led to a reduction in medications. The patients who exercised the most improved the most.

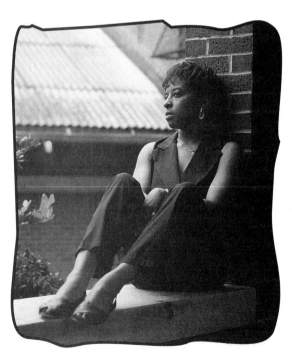

Depression can range from a mild form of blues to severe clinical depression.

Summary

♦ Cancer is the second leading cause of death in the U. S.

♦ Cancer is characterized by abnormal and uncontrollable cellular growth.

♦ Oncogenes are cancerous genes.

♦ Exercise helps to prevent cancer by reducing body fat, stimulating the immune system, and increasing the transit of food through the digestive system.

♦ Osteoporosis is a "silent" disease characterized by the gradual loss of bone mass.

♦ Women are affected by osteoporosis more often and at an earlier age than men.

♦ Risk factors for osteoporosis include age, gender, heredity, lack of physical activity, cigarette smoking, and insufficient calcium intake.

♦ Osteoporosis is treatable but not curable.

♦ Weight-bearing aerobic exercises and weight-training exercise are best for developing and maintaining the skeletal system.

♦ Osteoarthritis is the result of wear of the cartilage between joints.

♦ The major cause of osteoarthritis is obesity.

♦ Exercise alleviates osteoarthritis by lubricating and nourishing the joints.

♦ Nonweight-bearing exercises, such as water sports and activities, can be used if land-based weight-bearing exercises cause pain.

♦ Asthma-related deaths in the United States number more than 5000 annually.

♦ The American Academy of Allergy and Immunology encourages asthmatics to exercise regularly.

♦ Exercised-induced asthma occurs from the loss of respiratory heat and water resulting from high breathing rates.

♦ Of the many forms of exercise, swimming and other water activities are the least asthmogenic.

- Stress is the nonspecific response of the human organism to any demand, positive or negative, that it encounters.

- The individual's response or reaction to a stressor rather than the stressor itself, determines its impact.

- Acute stress is situational and of short duration, whereas chronic stress is long-term and potentially harmful.

- Physically fit people have a reduced response to stress, recover more rapidly, and are less vulnerable to stress-related diseases.

- Physically fit people develop a more robust immune system, have higher levels of endorphins, and have lower circulating catecholamine levels.

- Clinical depression, prolonged sadness that persists beyond a reasonable time, responds to regular exercise.

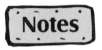
Notes

1. *Cancer Facts and Figures — 1997* (Atlanta: American Cancer Society, 1997).

2. M. A. Whaley and L. A. Kaminsky, "Epidemiology of Physical Activity, Physical Fitness, and Selected Chronic Diseases," *ACSM's Resource Manual for Guidelines for Exercise Testing and Prescription*, 3d edition, edited by J. L. Roitman (Baltimore: Williams and Wilkins, 1998).

3. I-M Lee, C. C. Hsieh, and R. S. Paffenbarger, "Exercise Intensity and Longevity in Men: The Harvard Alumni Health Study," *Journal of the American Medical Association*, 273 (April 19, 1995), 1179–1184.

4. S. N. Blair et al., "Changes in Physical Fitness and All-Cause Mortality," *Journal of the American Medical Association*, 273 (April 12, 1995), 1093–1098.

5. *Cancer Facts and Figures — 1997*.

6. "Exercise Wards Off Breast Cancer," *Tufts University Health and Nutrition Letter*, 15:5 (July, 1997), 6.

7. *Cancer Facts and Figures — 1997*.

8. I-M Lee, "Exercise and Physical Health: Cancer and Immune Function," *Research Quarterly for Exercise and Sport*, 66:4 (Dec. 1995), 286–291.

9. *Cancer Facts and Figures — 1997*.

10. D. C. Nieman, *Exercise Testing and Prescription: A Health-Related Approach* (Mountain View, CA: Mayfield, 1999).

11. *Osteoporosis: A Harvard Health Publications Special Report* (Boston: President and Fellows of Harvard College, July, 1997).

12. F. D. Wolinsky, J. F. Fitzgerald, and T. E. Stump, "The Effect of Hip Fracture on Mortality, Hospitalization, and Functional Status: A Prospective Study," *American Journal of Public Health*, 87 (1997) 398–403.

13. A. L. Fassler and J. P. Bonjour, "Osteoporosis as a Pediatric Problem," *Pediatrics Clinics of North America*, 42 (1995) 811–824.

14. J. M. Shaw and K. A. Witzke, "Exercise for Skeletal Health and Osteoporosis Prevention," *ACSM's Resource Manual for Guidelines for Exercise Testing and Prescription*.

15. ACSM, "Position Stand: Osteoporosis and Exercise," *Medicine and Science in Sports and Exercise*, 27:4 (1995), i–vii.

16. Shaw and Witzke.

17. "Exercise and Arthritis: The Importance of a Regular Program," *University of California at Berkeley Wellness Letter*, 10 (April 1994), 6.

18. D. T. Felson, "Obesity and Knee Osteoarthritis: The Framingham Study," *Annals of Internal Medicine* 109 (1988), 18.

19. D. T. Felson, "Weight and Osteoarthritis," *American Journal of Clinical Nutrition*, 63 (Suppl) (1996), 4305–4325.

20. C. X. Bryant, J. A. Peterson, and J. E. Graves, "Muscular Strength and Endurance," *ACSM's Resource Manual for Guidelines for Exercise Testing and Prescription*.

21. F. S. Sanders, "Exercise Induced Asthma in Athletes," *ACSM Certified News* 7:3 (Dec. 1997), 1–3.

22. C. C. W. Hsia, "Pathophysiology of Lung Disease," *ACSM's Resource Manual for Guidelines for Exercise Testing and Prescription.*

23. D. Mahler, "Exercise-Induced Asthma," *Medicine and Science in Sports and Exercise*, 25 (May, 1993), 554.

24. Sanders.

25. Adapted from R. Rosato, *Fitness For Wellness — The Physical Connection* (St. Paul: West Publishing, 1994).

26. Nieman.

Nutrition
for Active People

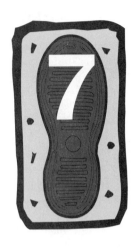

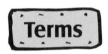

Adipose

Amino acids

Anabolism

Android obesity

Antioxidant

Basal metabolic rate (BMR)

Body mass index (BMI)

Catabolism

DNA

Diuretics

Electrolytes

Essential fat

Free radicals

Gynoid obesity

Homeostasis

Hydrogenation

Insoluble fiber

Lipids

Macronutrients

Metabolism

Micronutrients

Morbidity

Mortality

Nutrient-dense

Nutrients

Overfat

Overweight

Oxidation

Percent body fat

Percent daily value

Phytochemicals

Recommended
dietary allowance (RDA)

Resting metabolic rate
(RMR)

Skinfold

Soluble fiber

Storage fat

Transfatty acids

Triglycerides

Waist/hip ratio (WHR)

Weight cycling

Nutrition goes hand-in-hand with exercise in promoting health and well-being. In this chapter we will explore how the body uses the various nutrients, particularly the energy nutrients that provide fuel for bodily activity. The discussion encompasses weight control for both overweight and underweight people, including techniques for measuring body composition.

This chapter covers the basics of a nutritious diet and the effects of diet and exercise on weight control. The basic **nutrients** that allow the body to perform its many functions are carbohydrates, fats, protein, vitamins, minerals, and water. They provide fuel for muscle contraction, maintain and repair body tissues, regulate chemical reactions at the cellular level, transmit neural impulses, and provide for the growth and reproduction of cells.

This chapter also addresses the roles of nutrition and exercise in weight control. Selected techniques for measuring overweight and overfat are included.

BASIC NUTRITION

Metabolism is the sum total of chemical reactions by which the energy liberated from food is made available to the body. Two processes are involved:

1. Anabolism: incorporating substances into new tissues or storing them in some form for later use,

2. Catabolism: breaking down complex materials to simpler ones to release energy for muscular contraction.

Catabolism occurs when food is combined with oxygen. This process of **oxidation** transforms food materials into heat or mechanical energy. The energy value of food is expressed in calories. In this text we are using the term kcal, the amount of heat needed to increase the temperature of 1 kilogram of water (slightly more than one quart) by 1 degree centigrade. This sometimes is referred to as the nutritionist's calorie in that it is the unit commonly used to assign the caloric value to food.

Food Guide Pyramid

In 1992 the U. S. Department of Agriculture released the Food Guide Pyramid, Figure 7.1, which replaced the basic four food groups and is a significant step forward in directing the nation's attention toward healthier eating. From a health perspective, the foods that a person should eat in the greatest quantities are the breads, cereals, pastas, fruits, and vegetables, located at the base of the pyramid. The least desirable foods (fats, oils, and sweets) are located at the apex. Each level is accompanied by the suggested number of daily servings.

Although the Food Guide Pyramid is a useful guide, it has some deficiencies, among them:

1. It gives no indication of how large a serving should be.

2. Dry beans should not be in the third level with meat because of the significant difference in fat content between the two.

3. It makes no mention of skim milk dairy products.

4. It does not differentiate saturated and unsaturated fats.

Barring these criticisms, it is a worthy guide.

Subsequent to development of the Food Guide Pyramid (FGP), the federal government stepped in and standardized serving sizes that reflect the amounts that people actually eat.[1] Before then, manufacturers were allowed to establish the serving sizes for their products. Examples of serving sizes for the various categories are included in Figure 7.1.

Nutrition Facts Food Label

Since May 1994, all processed foods must display the new food label mandated by the federal government. These are a substantial improvement over the old ones in that they facilitate comparison of foods based on nutritional quantity and quality. The upper half of the new label contains the nutritional information related specifically to the food in the package. The lower half is for reference purposes and is constant for all food products.

The upper half of the label provides the **percent daily value** for six important nutrients. The sample food label in Figure 7.2 indicates that the total fat in this specific food represents 5% of the daily allowance, and the sodium (salt) content of this item is 13% of the daily allowance. The information on the upper half of the label can assist consumers in planning their daily menu without exceeding the nutritional recommendations for a given day. It also allows them to select the best foods by comparison of caloric content as well as nutrient content.

The lower half provides the upper limit for selected nutrients for diets consisting of either 2000 kcals or 2500 kcals. The person should adjust these values in accordance with the total calorie intake.

Food Guide Pyramid
A Guide to Daily Food Choices

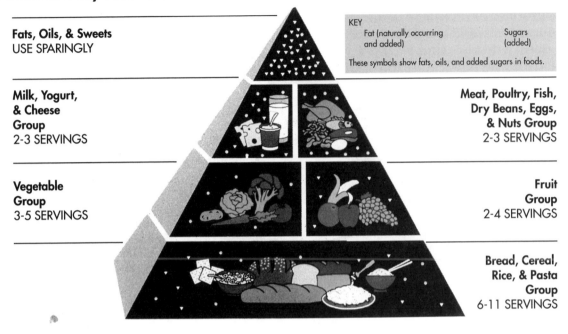

Fats, Oils, & Sweets
USE SPARINGLY

KEY
Fat (naturally occurring and added)   Sugars (added)

These symbols show fats, oils, and added sugars in foods.

Milk, Yogurt, & Cheese Group
2-3 SERVINGS

Meat, Poultry, Fish, Dry Beans, Eggs, & Nuts Group
2-3 SERVINGS

Vegetable Group
3-5 SERVINGS

Fruit Group
2-4 SERVINGS

Bread, Cereal, Rice, & Pasta Group
6-11 SERVINGS

What counts as a serving?

Grain Products Group (bread, cereal, rice, and pasta)
- 1 slice of bread
- 1 ounce of ready-to-eat cereal
- ½ cup of cooked cereal, rice, or pasta

Vegetable Group
- 1 cup of raw leafy vegetables
- ½ cup of other vegetables — cooked or chopped raw
- ¾ cup of vegetable juice

Fruit Group
- 1 medium apple, banana, orange
- ½ cup of chopped, cooked, or canned fruit
- ¾ cup of fruit juice

Milk Group (milk, yogurt, and cheese)
- 1 cup of milk or yogurt
- 1½ ounces of natural cheese
- 2 ounces of processed cheese

Meat and Beans Group (meat, poultry, fish, dry beans, eggs, and nuts)
- 2–3 ounces of cooked lean meat, poultry, or fish
- ½ cup of cooked dry beans or 1 egg counts as 1 ounce of lean meat. 2 tablespoons of peanut butter or ⅓ cup of nuts count as 1 ounce of meat.

*Some foods fit into more than one group. Dry beans, peas, and lentils can be counted as servings either in the meat and beans group or the vegetable group. These "crossover" foods can be counted as servings from either one or the other group, but not both.

Source: U. S. Dept. of Agriculture and U. S. Dept. of Health and Human Services, *Nutrition and Your Health: Dietary Guidelines for Americans*, (Washington DC: U. S. Government Printing Office, 1996). (Home and Garden Bulletin No. 232).

Figure 7.1   Food Guide Pyramid: A guide to daily food choices.

The Calorie-Containing Nutrients

The nutrients are classified into six categories: carbohydrates, fats, proteins, vitamins, minerals, and water. The first three are referred to as the "energy nutrients," and the last three as the "regulatory nutrients."

Nutrition facts
Serving size 1/2 cup (114 g)
Servings per container 4

Amount per serving

Calories 90   Calories from fat 30

	Percent Daily Value *
Total fat 3 g	5%
Saturated fat 0 g	0%
Cholesterol 0 mg	0%
Sodium 30 mg	13%
Total carbohydrate 13 g	4%
Dietary fiber 3 g	12%
Sugars 3 g	
Protein 3 g	

Vitamin A	80%	Vitamin C	60%
Calcium	4%	Iron	4%

*Percent Daily Values are based on a 2,000 calorie diet. Your daily values may be higher or lower depending on your calorie needs:

		Calories	2,000	2,500
Total fat	Less than		65 g	80 g
Saturated fat	Less than		20 g	25 g
Cholesterol	Less than		300 mg	300 mg
Sodium	Less than		2,400 mg	2,400 mg
Total carbohydrate			300 g	375 g
Fiber			25 g	30 g

Calories per gram:
Fat 9   Carbohydrates 4   Protein 4.

Figure 7.2 Sample new food label.

Carbohydrates

Carbohydrates are organic compounds composed of one or more sugars (saccharides) that are derived from plants. Carbohydrates consist of monosaccharides (simple sugars), disaccharides (combination of two simple sugars), and polysaccharides (the joining of three or more simple sugars to form starch and glycogen).

Examples of simple sugars are table sugar, corn syrup, molasses, and honey. People in the United States, active and inactive alike, consume too much of these substances. Simple sugar consumption has risen steadily for the last decade. The average consumption in 1986 was 128 pounds per person. By 1996, sugar consumption had increased to 152 pounds per person.[2] Most of the sugar intake in the United States is hidden in processed foods, the biggest offender of which is soft drinks. Americans spent $54 billion on soft drinks in 1997.[3] We currently are consuming soft drinks at a rate double that of milk and nearly six times that of fruit juices. A 12-ounce can of non-diet cola has about 10 teaspoons of sugar and 150 calories. Large amounts of sugar also are added to ice cream, candy, pastries, canned meats, canned soups and vegetables, and other canned products. Simple sugars are considered "empty calories," as the 112 calories per ounce they produce have little, if any, nutritional value.

Many authorities believe the excessive consumption of simple sugars leads to obesity, Type II diabetes, elevated cholesterol, heart disease, and dental caries, although the bulk of the evidence does not support most of these assumptions.[4] According to the American Dietetic Association, sugar has been erroneously indicted as the cause of a number of health problems.[5] Sugar is not an independent risk factor for any disease, except in the case of a few rare heredity disorders. For people who are insulin-resistant, however, sugar consumption increases the risk for heart disease by raising blood triglyceride levels. Also, it is a major cause of tooth decay. Sugar should constitute less than 10% of the total calories (see Table 7.1).

The bulk of carbohydrates consumed should come from the complex form. These include

Table 7.1 Consumption of the Three Energy Nutrients —
Current and Recommended

Food Category	Current Consumption (% of total kcals)	Recommended Consumption (% of total kcals)
Carbohydrates	48% a. 1/2 sugar b. 1/2 complex carbohydrates	55% a. < 10% sugar * b. 45% complex carbohydrates
Fat	34% a. 12% saturated b. 22% unsaturated c. 10% polyunsaturated	a. < 10% saturated b. 10% monounsaturated
Protein	15%	15%

* < means less than

Source: Data compiled by the American Heart Association, the American Dietetic Association, and found in the *Nutrition and Diet Therapy Dictionary.*

starch and several forms of fiber. The complex carbohydrates are **nutrient-dense** for the number of calories they contain. This category of food is precisely what weight- and health-conscious people need. Today's dictum for health and weight control is to "lower the fat content of the diet." Increasing the intake of complex carbohydrates is a painless way to do this. Starchy foods — grains, legumes, tubers, and pastas — are both healthy and tasty. All starches come from plant foods, most of which contain only trace amounts of fat. Exceptions include olives, avocados, nuts, seeds, and coconuts, which contain substantial amounts of fat and therefore should be consumed in moderation.

A diet high in plant foods also will be high in fiber. Processing and refining plant products diminishes the quantity of fiber significantly, if not totally. Dietary fiber is of two types: soluble, which dissolves in hot water, and insoluble, which does not dissolve. Both are beneficial to health but in different ways. Both are indigestible polysaccharides found in the stems, leaves, and seeds of plants.

Soluble fiber adds bulk to the stomach contents. This slows stomach emptying and prolongs the sense of feeling full. This is especially good for weight watchers. Soluble fiber also lowers blood cholesterol levels. Reducing body weight and cholesterol lower the risk for cardiovascular disease.

Insoluble fiber adds bulk to the contents of the intestines, thereby accelerating the passage of food through the digestive tract. This has several healthy effects:

1. It decreases the time that body tissue is exposed to toxins and carcinogenic substances, thereby providing some protection against colon cancer.

2. It prevents or alleviates constipation.

3. It stimulates muscle tone in the intestinal walls, which increases resistance to diverticulosis (a condition of saclike swellings in the intestinal wall).

Most plants contain some of both types of fiber. Good sources of fiber are listed in Table 7.2.

When oxidized, carbohydrates yield approximately 4 calories per gram. Because they are oxygen-rich, carbohydrates constitute the most efficient source of fuel. They are the major energy supplier in high-intensity work of short duration and in exercise of a vigorous nature for up to 60 to 90 minutes.

Foods high in carbohydrates promote the storage of glycogen (the stored form of sugar) in the liver and muscles. Increasing the storage of glycogen enhances aerobic performance of long duration such as marathon running and long-distance cycling. People who do not run such long distances should consume a diet rich in complex carbohydrates primarily because it is a healthy way to eat. Active adults should consume about 45% of their calories in the form of complex carbohydrates and no more than 10% in the form of simple sugars. By contrast, people who train for and compete in prolonged endurance

Table 7.2   Selected Sources of Fiber

Sources	Dietary Fiber (grams)	Sources	Dietary Fiber (grams)
1. Cereals		Potato, baked (1 medium)	3.8
Kellogg's All-Bran Extra Fiber (½ cup)	15	Carrots (1 raw; ½ cup cooked)	2.3
General Mills Fiber one (½ cup)	14	Collards	2.2
Kellogg's All-Bran (½ cup)	10	Asparagus	2.1
100% Bran (½ cup)	8.4	Green beans	2.1
All Bran (½ cup)	8.5	Broccoli	2.0
Bran Buds (⅓ cup)	7.9	Spinach	2.0
Bran Chex (⅔ cup)	4.6	Turnips	1.7
Corn Bran (⅔ cup)	5.4	Mushrooms (raw)	0.9
Cracklin' Oat Bran (⅓ cup)	4.3	Summer squash	0.7
Bran Flakes (¾ cup)	4.0	Lettuce (raw)	0.3
Oatmeal, cooked (1 cup)	2.2	5. Fruits	
2. Grains (1 ounce)		Blackberries (½ cup)	4.5
Brown rice, cooked (½ cup)	2.4	Prunes, dried (3)	3.7
Millet, cooked (½ cup)	1.8	Apples with skin (1)	2.6
Whole wheat bread (1 slice)	1.0	Banana (1 medium)	2.0
Spaghetti, cooked (½ cup)	0.8	Strawberries (¾ cup)	2.0
White bread (1 slice)	0.6	Grapefruit (½ med)	1.7
White rice, cooked (½ cup)	0.1	Peach (1 med)	1.6
3. Legumes (½ cup)		Cantaloupe (¼ small)	1.4
Kidney beans	5.8	Raisins (2 tablespoons)	1.3
Pinto beans	5.3	Orange (1 small)	1.2
Split peas	5.1	Grapes (12)	0.5
White beans	5.0		
Lima beans	4.9		
4. Vegetables (½ cup)			
Sweet potato (1 large)	4.2		
Peas	4.1		
Brussels sprouts	3.9		
Corn	3.9		

Source: Adapted from *Plant Fiber in Foods* by J. Anderson (Lexington, KY: HFC Diabetes Research Foundation, 1986); *Nutrition Action Health-letter* (April 1986); and E. Lanza and R. R. Butram, "A Critical Review of Food Fiber Analysis and Data," *Journal of the American Dietetic Association*, 86 (1986), 732.

events should consume 65% to 70% of their calories from the carbohydrate group.

Fats

Fats are energy-dense organic compounds that yield approximately 9 calories per gram. They have a relatively low oxygen content when compared to carbohydrates and, consequently, are not as efficient as sources of fuel. More than twice the amount of oxygen is required to liberate energy from fat than from carbohydrates. Meanwhile, we store at least 50 times more energy in the form of fat than carbohydrates. A pound of fat as it is stored in the body contains 3500 kcals.

The most abundant of the fats, or **lipids**, are the **triglycerides**. Triglycerides make-up at least 98% of the fat we consume as well as the fat we store. Triglycerides are composed of three fatty acids attached to a molecule of glycerol. As

depicted in Figure 7.3, fatty acids are saturated when all of the bonds between the carbon atoms are single bonds (a). Monounsaturated fatty acids have one double bond between carbon atoms (b). Polyunsaturated fatty acids have two or more double bonds between the carbon atoms (c).

The major sources of saturated fats are animal flesh, dairy products, and tropical oils (coconut and palm kernel oils). Saturated fats have a high melting point and solidify at room temperature. Bacon or sausage grease that stands at room temperature will solidify, signifying that it is saturated. Monounsaturated and polyunsaturated fats remain liquid at room temperature. Some food sources that are high in monounsaturated fats are avocados, canola oil, cashew nuts, olives, olive oil, peanuts, peanut oil, and peanut butter. Polyunsaturated fats are found in almonds, corn oil, cottonseed oil, filbert nuts, fish, pecans, safflower oil, sunflower oil, soybean oil,

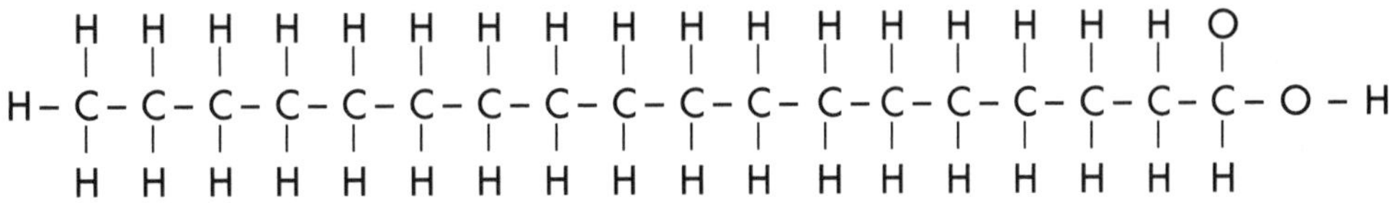

(a) Saturated fatty acid — no double bonds: all carbons are occupied.

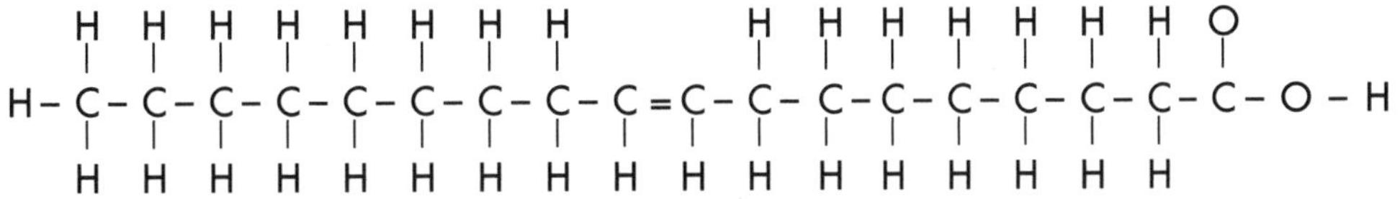

(b) Monounsaturated fatty acid — one double bond; two hydrogens missing at that site.

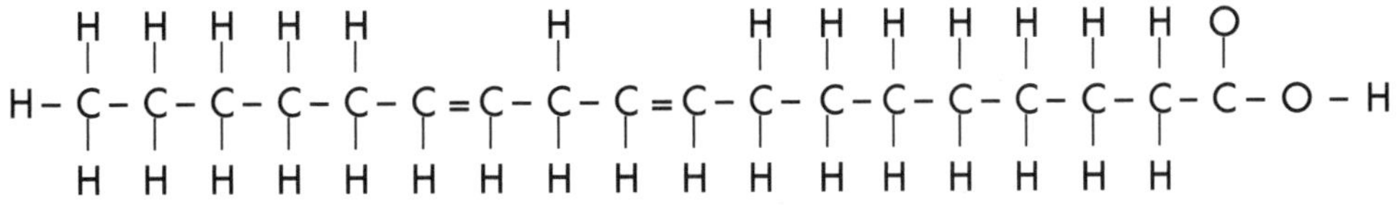

(c) Polyunsaturated fatty acid — two double bonds; four hydrogen missing at the site

Figure 7.3 Different types of fatty acids.

and walnuts. Some sources of plant-derived cooking oils appear in Table 7.3.

Fatty acids derived from fish, especially cold-water fish, are different from those found in vegetables and vegetable oils. The fatty acids in fish are Omega-3 fatty acids, and those found in vegetables are primarily Omega-6 fatty acids. Omega-3 fatty acids protect the heart and its blood vessels by decreasing the likelihood that the blood platelets will stick to each other. This in turn reduces plaque build-up, clot formation, and spasms in the arteries.[6]

Transfatty acids

Unsaturated fats should be refrigerated to keep them from becoming rancid. They are vulnerable to spoilage when they are left to stand at room temperature because oxygen attacks those points in the chain that are unoccupied by hydrogen. To counteract spoilage, the food industry adds hydrogen to some of the free bonds through the process of **hydrogenation**. The fat then loses its polyunsaturated characteristics as well its health benefits. Hydrogenation converts many double bonds to single bonds. The end product is the conversion of unsaturated fatty acids to **transfatty acids**. Margarine is one of the major sources of transfatty acids in the U.S. diet. In addition, transfatty acids are found in cookies, crackers, pies, cakes, peanut butter, fast-food fried chicken, french fries, fish — and this is just a partial list. Approximately 5% to 10% of the fat in the average U.S. diet is transfat.[7]

Vegetable oils are liquid and must be made more saturated if they are to be solidified into margarine. The harder the product (stick margarine) — versus softer margarines (tub and squeeze bottle) — the greater is the effect of hydrogenation. The question to be answered is: Does the conversion of unsaturated fatty acids to transfatty acids result in an unhealthy product? Some evidence indicates that transfatty acids have an effect similar to the saturated fats — that is, they raise the blood level of harmful LDL cholesterol.[8] Unfortunately, the new food labels do not record the grams of transfatty acids found in processed foods.

Eating a fat-free diet is virtually impossible and definitely unhealthy. The human body requires some fat. Two fatty acids, in fact, are

---

Table 7.3 Some Sources of Plant-Derived Cooking Oils

Type of Oil (grams)	Monounsaturated (grams)	Polyunsaturated (grams)	Saturated
Best Sources			
Almond	10	2	1
Canola	8	4	1
Olive	10	1	2
Good Sources			
Corn	3	8	2
Cottonseed	2	7	4
Safflower	2	10	1
Sesame	5	6	2
Soybean	3	8	2
Sunflower	3	9	1

Note: 1 gram = $1/28$ ounce.

essential. They must be obtained through the diet because they cannot be manufactured from other substances in the body. Both are polyunsaturated fatty acids that are widely distributed in plant and fish oils.

1. *Linoleic acid*, an Omega-6 fatty acid found in plants,

2. *Linolenic fatty acid*, an Omega-3 fatty acid, found primarily in fish.

Proteins

Protein is an essential nutrient that yields approximately 4 calories per gram. Its energy is liberated for building and repairing body tissues; forming enzymes, hormones, antibodies, and hemoglobin; transporting fats and other nutrients through the blood; maintaining the acid-base balance in tissue fluids; and supplying energy for muscular work when there is a shortage of carbohydrates and fat.

Proteins are complex chemical structures containing carbon, oxygen, hydrogen, and nitrogen. These elements are combined into chains of different structures called amino acids. The proteins of all living tissue consist of 20 different **amino acids**. Two other rare amino acids have been identified but are found in very few proteins. Nine of the amino acids are considered *essential* because the body cannot manufacture

them and they can be obtained only through the diet. Complete proteins — those containing all the essential amino acids — are found in meat, fish, poultry, and dairy products. The proteins found in vegetables and cereal grains generally do not contain all of the essential amino acids, but complementary foods from these two groups may be selected so that one supplies the amino acids missing in the other. Table 7.4 provides combinations of food that together provide complete proteins.

Legumes, such as kidney and lima beans, black-eyed peas, garden peas, lentils, and soybeans, are excellent sources of proteins. Although their protein is not quite the caliber of meat protein, they are rich in other healthy nutrients such as B vitamins, and they are low in fat.

Daily protein requirements vary according to age. Infants require about 2.2 grams of protein per kilogram of body weight to support growth. Adolescents require 1.0 gram per kilogram. Adults need 0.8 gram per kilogram.

The typical U.S. diet contains more than adequate protein. Consuming more than 15% of the total calories in the form of protein seems to have no advantage. One of the major problems associated with excessive protein intake is that it is usually accomplished by increasing the consumption of animal products, which also are high in saturated fat. The increased consumption could displace fiber in the diet, and the two

Table 7.4 Vegetable Combinations That Provide Complete Proteins

Categories of Foods	Examples
Beans/wheat	Baked beans and brown bread
Beans/rice	Refried beans and rice
Dry peas/rye	Split pea soup and rye bread
Peanut butter/wheat	Peanut butter sandwich on whole wheat or whole grain bread
Cornmeal/beans	Cornbread and kidney beans
Legumes/rice	Black-eyed peas and rice
Beans/corn	Pinto beans and cornbread
Legumes/corn	Black-eyed peas and cornbread

Adapted from *The Vegetarian Athlete* by A. C. Grandjeans 15 (1987), 191.

together can lead to a host of immediate and long-term problems.

The average daily consumption of protein by adults in the United States is about 16% of total calories — well above the requirement. For example, a 154-pound person requires 56 grams of protein each day. If this person is consuming 2500 kcals/day with a typical protein intake of 15%, this person actually is consuming 94 grams of protein. These figures come from the following:

1. Protein requirement is calculated as follows:
   a. Convert body weight in pounds to kilograms (kg)
      154 ÷ 2.2 = 70 kg
   b. 70 kg × .8 grams = 56 grams/day
2. Actual consumption is calculated as follows:
   a. 2500 kcals/day
      × .15
      375 kcals of protein
   b. 1 gram of protein yields 4 kcals; therefore
      375 kcals ÷ 4 = 94 grams/protein
   c. The difference between protein consumed and protein required is:
      94 g consumed
      −56 g required
      38 extra grams of protein

Many people — competitors and noncompetitors alike — who are striving to develop strength and power take amino acid supplements to build larger and more powerful muscles. Selected amino acids do not build larger muscles. Only exercise can do that. Nevertheless, these and other unfounded notions proliferate among uninformed participants who are constantly attempting to enhance their performance with substances that might give them an edge beyond that they achieve through training.

Current evidence indicates that long-distance, endurance-type athletes and weightlifters and bodybuilders have the greatest need for protein — 1.5 to 1.6 grams of protein for every kilogram of body weight.[9] Even if this proves to be correct,

protein supplements are not necessary, as most athletes consume more than this amount from their food intake.

Suppose a 145-pound marathon runner consumes 4,800 kcals/day. His protein intake represents 15% of his total calories. How many grams of protein does he consume, and how many does he actually need if his requirement is 1½ times the normal amount for adults?

1. Convert body weight in pounds to kilograms (kg)
   145 lbs. ÷ 2.2 = 66 kg
2. 4800 kcals consumed
   × .15 percentage of protein in diet
   720 kcals/protein
3. 1 gram of protein yields 4 kcals; therefore,
   720 ÷ 4 = 180 grams protein intake
4. Protein required is 1.6 grams per kg of body weight
   66 kg
   × 1.6
   105.6 grams
5. Difference between protein consumed and protein required:
   180 consumed
   −106 needed
   74 grams of extra protein

In light of this example, protein supplementation or amino acid supplements are unnecessary and a waste of money.

The Non-Calorie-Containing Nutrients

The regulatory nutrients, which contain no calories, are vitamins, minerals, and water.

Vitamins

Vitamins are organic compounds found in small quantities in most foods. All vitamins are either fat-soluble or water-soluble. The fat-soluble vitamins (A, D, E, and K) are stored in the liver and fatty tissues until they are needed.

The water-soluble vitamins (C and the B complex group) are not stored for any appreciable length of time and must be replenished daily.

Vitamins function as coenzymes that promote the many chemical reactions in the body around the clock. Because vitamin deficiencies result in a variety of diseases and adequate daily intake is necessary, the **recommended dietary allowance (RDA)** for most vitamins has been established. Although these amounts are needed to prevent vitamin deficiency diseases, they do not represent optimal values. Today, the interest in vitamins by the scientific community goes beyond that. For instance, substantial research efforts currently are attempting to clarify the role of selected **antioxidant** vitamins (C, E, and beta-carotene) in preventing cardiovascular disease and cancer. The early evidence is promising, and taking these vitamins in larger amounts than recommended appear to be safe.

The antioxidant vitamins protect the body from the harmful effects of **free radicals** (oxidants). Free radicals are byproducts of oxidation. Because the cells continuously use oxygen, free radicals are being produced constantly. Simultaneously, free radicals are generated by cigarette smoke, radiation from the sun and other sources, alcohol, heat, and environmental pollutants.

If free radicals are not neutralized immediately, they damage the cells and their **DNA** (the master blueprint for cellular function). Researchers estimate that each DNA of the approximately 60 trillion cells in the body takes "a hit from free radicals every 10 seconds."[10] Over the course of a lifetime, some of the cellular damage inflicted by free radicals goes unrepaired. The cumulative damage can result in the development of cancer, heart disease, cataracts, and rheumatoid arthritis. Free radicals also have been implicated as an agent that promotes aging.

The antioxidant vitamins protect the cells from the damaging effects of free radicals. Many authorities, but not all, recommend taking 500 milligrams (mg) of vitamin C and 400 international units (IU) of vitamin E daily to neutralize the free radicals. All authorities agree, however, that we should obtain antioxidants by increasing our consumption of fruits, vegetables, and whole grains. Eating these antioxidant-rich foods provides another advantage: They contain **phytochemicals**, which are unique to plant foods. There are literally hundreds, maybe thousands, of phytochemicals. The research that has identified these elements along with their potential health benefits is in the earliest stages of development. Thus far, the phytochemicals likely are involved in the prevention of cancer, heart disease, and other chronic diseases. Continuing research will provide more answers in the next few years.

Unusually large doses (megadoses) of any vitamin are potentially hazardous. People who supplement heavily may suffer vitamin toxicity, particularly from overindulgence in the fat-soluble group. When vitamins are taken in very large amounts, they cease to function as vitamins and begin to act like drugs. Also, large doses interfere with or disrupt the action of other nutrients. Tables 7.5 and 7.6 list some problems associated with vitamin megadoses.

Are synthetic vitamin supplements inferior to natural vitamin supplements? Promoters of vitamin products that come from natural sources adamantly proclaim that this is so but in reality the synthetic and natural supplements are

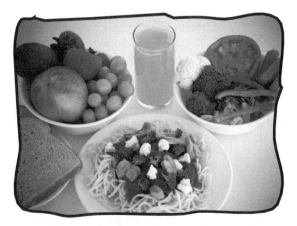

The experts agree that people should obtain antioxidants by eating more fruits, vegetables, and whole grains.

Active people tend to get more vitamins in their diet than sedentary people do because active people consume more calories than their less active counterparts. If you are concerned about not getting enough vitamins in your diet but are unwilling to make appropriate dietary changes, a one-a-day brand supplemented by extra C and E should suffice.

chemically equivalent and the body cannot tell them apart. Vitamin E is an exception. Natural vitamin E in supplement form is absorbed more easily than its synthetic counterpart. If a person takes 400 IU of vitamin E, it really doesn't matter whether the vitamin is natural or synthetic because the body will absorb and use more than enough.

Minerals

Minerals are inorganic substances that exist freely in nature. They are found in the earth's soil and water, and they pervade some of the earth's vegetation. Minerals maintain or regulate physiological processes such as muscle contraction, normal heart rhythm, body water supplies,

Table 7.5 Toxic Symptoms of Fat-Soluble Vitamins

Vitamin (U.S. RDA)	Sources	Toxic Symptoms
Vitamin A *(1000 mg)	fortified milk and margarine, cream, cheese, butter, eggs, liver, spinach and other dark leafy greens, broccoli, apricots, peaches, cantaloupe, squash, carrots, sweet potatoes, pumpkin	red blood cell breakage, nosebleeds, abdominal cramps, nausea, diarrhea, weight loss, blurred vision, irritability, loss of appetite, bone pain, dry skin, rashes, hair loss, cessation of menstruation, growth retardation
Vitamin D **(400 IU)	self-synthesis with sunlight, fortified milk, fortified margarine, eggs, liver, fish	elevated blood calcium, constipation, weight loss, irritability, weakness, nausea, kidney stones, mental and physical retardation
Vitamin E (30 IU)	vegetable oils, green leafy vegetables, wheat germ, whole-grain products, butter, liver, egg yolk, milk fat, nuts, seeds	interference with anticlotting medication, general discomfort
Vitamin K (no U.S. RDA)	bacterial synthesis in digestive tract, liver, green leafy and cruciferous vegetables, milk	interference with anticlotting medication; may cause jaundice

*mg = micrograms
** IU = international units

Table 7.6 Toxic Symptoms of Water-Soluble Vitamins

Vitamin (U.S. RDA)	Sources	Toxic Symptoms
Thiamin B₁ *(1.5 mg)	meat, pork, liver, fish, poultry, whole-grain and enriched breads, cereals, pasta, nuts, legumes, wheat germ, oats	rapid pulse, weakness, headaches, insomnia, irritability
Riboflavin B₂ (1.7 mg)	milk, dark green vegetables, yogurt, cottage cheese, liver, meat, whole-grain or enriched breads and cereals	none reported, but an excess of any of the B vitamins could cause a deficiency of the others
Niacin B₃ (20 mg)	meat, eggs, poultry, fish, milk, whole-grain and enriched breads and cereals, nuts, legumes, peanuts, nutritional yeast, all protein foods	flushing, nausea, headaches, cramps, ulcer irritation, heartburn, abnormal liver function, low blood pressure
Vitamin B₆ (2.0 mg)	meat, poultry, fish, shellfish, legumes, whole-grain products, green leafy vegetables, bananas	depression, fatigue, irritability, headaches, numbness, damage to nerves, difficulty walking
Folcain (Folic acid) (400 micrograms)	green leafy vegetables, organ meats, legumes, seeds	diarrhea, insomnia, irritability; could mask a vitamin B₁₂ deficiency
Vitamin B₁₂ **(cobalamin) (3 g)	animal products: meats, fish, poultry, shellfish, milk, cheese, eggs, nutritional yeast	none reported
Pantothenic acid (10 mg)	widespread in foods	occasional diarrhea
Biotin (300 g)	widespread in foods	none reported
Vitamin C (Ascorbic acid) (60 mg)	citrus fruits, cruciferous vegetables, tomatoes, potatoes, dark green vegetables, peppers, lettuce, cantaloupe, strawberries, mangos, papayas	nausea, abdominal cramps, diarrhea, breakdown of red blood cells in persons with certain genetic disorders: deficiency symptoms might appear at first upon withdrawal of high doses

* mg = micrograms
** g = grams

acid-base balance of the blood, and nerve impulse conduction. The major minerals are calcium, phosphorous, potassium, sulphur, sodium, chloride, and magnesium. They are classified as **macronutrients** because they occur in the body in quantities greater than 5 grams. The trace minerals, or **micronutrients**, number a dozen or more. The distinction between the major and trace minerals is one of quantity rather than importance. Deficiencies of either can have serious consequences.

Sodium, potassium, and chloride are the minerals lost primarily through perspiration. Sodium, the positive ion in sodium chloride (table salt), is one of the body's major **electrolytes** (ions that conduct electricity). Although Americans consume 3 to 4 grams of sodium daily, only 1.8 to 2.4 grams are recommended.[11] Approximately 70% of the salt consumed in the United States is in processed foods such as canned and instant soups, smoked meats and fish, cheeses, and deep-fried snacks. Salt is a cheap preservative and flavor enhancer. The labels on all canned and packaged foods indicate the amount of sodium the product contains. The other 30% of our salt intake comes from using the salt shaker and from naturally occurring salt in the foods we eat.

Sodium is found in the fluid outside of the cells, and potassium is found within cellular fluid. The temporary exchange of sodium and potassium across the cell's membrane permits the transmission of neural impulses and the contraction of muscles. Low potassium levels interfere with muscle-cell nutrition and lead to muscle weakness and fatigue. Potassium is essential to maintain the heartbeat.

Starvation and very low calorie diets for prolonged periods can produce sudden death from heart failure as potassium storage drops to critically low levels. Vomiting, diarrhea, and **diuretics** reduce potassium levels. Chronic physical activity that produces heavy sweating probably will not diminish potassium stores unless the diet is woefully lacking in this mineral. It is hard to reduce potassium stores because most foods contain potassium and it is easily replaced. Potassium is particularly abundant in citrus fruits and juices, bananas, dates, nuts, fresh vegetables, meat, and fish.

As with vitamins, mineral intake can be abused. Excess amounts of major and trace minerals produce a variety of symptoms, as shown in Tables 7.7 and 7.8.

Water

People can survive for a month or more without food, but a few days without water will result in death. Because all body processes and chemical reactions take place in a liquid medium, the body has to be fully hydrated, and people should make a special effort to replace water when it is lost. Under normal conditions, adults drink 1.2 to 1.4 liters of fluid each day. More is needed when the weather is hot and humid and when a person is physically active regardless of weather conditions.

Approximately 60% of the body's weight consists of water. Much of it is stored in the muscles, and some is stored in fat. By virtue of his larger muscle mass, the average male stores more water than the average female. Of the total amount of water, 62% is found in the intracellular compartment (water within the cells) and the remaining 38% is extracellular (water in the blood, lymph system, spinal cord fluid, saliva, and so on).

The water level in the body is maintained primarily by drinking fluids. Solid foods, too, contribute to water replenishment. Many foods — fruits, vegetables, and meats — contain large amounts of water. Even seemingly dry foods such as bread contain some water. Solid foods add water in another way: They contribute metabolic water, one of the byproducts of their breakdown to energy sources.

Most of the water lost is through urination. Small quantities are lost in feces and in exhaled air from the lungs. Insensible perspiration (that which is not visible) accounts for a considerable amount of water loss. Because exercise and hot, humid weather increase sweating, more water must be consumed during these times. Exercise in hot weather and water replacement guidelines were included in Chapter 4.

THE REDUCTION EQUATION: EXERCISE + SENSIBLE EATING = FAT CONTROL

Exercise is important in reducing body weight — specifically fat weight — while sparing or enhancing muscle tissue. Exercise uses calories, stimulates metabolism, and brings appetite in line with energy expenditure. On the other hand, dieting without exercise produces diminishing returns because metabolism slows down as caloric needs decrease. After a few weeks of dieting, the body goes into a survival mode and adapts to the reduced caloric intake. The diet becomes less effective, and continued weight loss is more difficult to accomplish.

Eventually, the diet ends, some or all of the old eating patterns are reestablished, and the lost weight is regained. If dieting becomes cyclical, each attempt at losing weight takes longer, but the lost weight is regained more quickly, and the likelihood of gaining additional weight increases. Very-low calorie diets should be avoided. Without supplementation, they cannot provide the required nutrients, and the effect of low-caloric intake on the metabolism is devastating.

Table 7.7 Toxic Symptoms of Major Minerals

Minerals (U.S. RDA)	Selected Sources	Toxic Symptoms
Calcium (1000 mg)	milk and milk products	excess calcium is excreted except in hormonal imbalance states
Phosphorus (1000 mg)	fish (with bones), tofu, greens, legumes, all animal tissues	excess phosphorus can cause relative deficiency of calcium
Magnesium (400 mg)	nuts, legumes, whole grains, dark green vegetables, seafoods, chocolate, cocoa	not known
Sodium (no U.S. RDA)	salt, soy sauce, moderate quantities in whole (unprocessed), foods, large amounts in processed foods	hypertension
Chloride (no U.S. RDA)	salt, soy sauce, moderate quantities in whole (unprocessed) foods, large amounts in processed foods	normally harmless (chlorine gas is a poison but evaporates from water), disturbed acid-base balance, vomiting
Potassium (no U.S. RDA)	all whole foods: meats, milk, fruits, vegetables, grains, legumes	causes muscular weakness, triggers vomiting; if given into a vein, can stop the heart
Sulfur (no U.S. RDA)	all protein-containing foods	would occur only if sulfur amino acids were eaten in excess; this (in animals) depresses growth

Effects of Exercise on Weight Control

The often neglected factor in a weight loss attempt is exercise. Exercise and diet are not mutually exclusive. They are complementary in that each has a unique contribution to make to weight loss. The role of exercise was addressed in 1985 at an international meeting on obesity. The unanimous consensus of the experts was that, if you are about to start a weight reduction program or if you are trying to maintain your present weight, success or failure can depend on whether you exercise.

Table 7.8 Toxic Symptoms of Trace Minerals

Minerals (U.S. RDA)	Selected Sources	Toxic Symptoms
Iodine (150 g)	iodized salt, seafood	very high intakes depress thyroid activity
Iron (18 mg)	red meats, fish, poultry, shellfish, eggs, legumes, dried fruits)	iron overload: infections, liver injury
Zinc (15 mg)	protein-containing foods: meats, fish, poultry, grains, vegetables	fever, nausea, vomiting, diarrhea
Copper (2 mg)	meats, drinking water	unknown except as part of a rare hereditary disease (Wilson's disease)
Fluoride (no U.S. RDA)	drinking water (if naturally fluoride-containing or fluoridated), tea, seafood	fluorosis (discoloration of teeth)
Selenium (no U.S. RDA)	seafood, meat, grains	disorders of digestive system
Chromium (no U.S. RDA)	meats, unrefined foods, fats, vegetable oils	unknown as a nutrition disorder; occupational exposures damage skin and kidneys
Molybdenum, (no U.S. RDA)	legumes, cereals, organ meats	enzyme inhibition
Manganese (no U.S. RDA)	widely distributed in foods	poisoning, nervous system disorders
Cobalt (no U.S. RDA)	meats, milk and milk products	unknown as a nutritional disorder

Exercise Burns Calories

The American College of Sports Medicine (ACSM) suggests that the minimal threshold of exercise for weight loss is 300 kcals per exercise session done at least three times a week (900 kcals), or 200 kcals per session performed at least four times a week (800 kcals).[12] These are minimum guidelines. You can turn to Tables 3.3, and 3.4 in Chapter 3 which contain the data that walkers and joggers can use to calculate the number of calories expended for a given body weight at a specific speed for a given amount of time. As fitness improves, the threshold for exercise should increase slowly so the weekly energy expenditure eventually will reach about 2000 kcals per week. This is considered optimal to enhance health and would require walking or jogging approximately 20 miles per week.

The kcals burned during recovery from exercise contribute marginally to weight loss. The body does not shut off completely after exercise; it recovers gradually. Extra kcals are burned during this period until the metabolism returns to a normal resting level. A rule of thumb is that 15 kcals are burned in recovery for every 100 kcals burned during exercise.[13] If 400 kcals are used during exercise, an extra 60 kcals will be used during the recovery period. Exercising at this level 5 days a week will result in approximately 4½ pounds lost in 1 year from the kcals burned in recovery from exercise. This is illustrated by the following:

$$60 \text{ kcals} \times 5 \text{ days} = 300 \text{ kcals/wk} \times 52 \text{ wks}$$

$$= \frac{15,600 \text{ kcals/yr}}{3500 \text{ kcals}} = 4.45 \text{ lbs}$$

Admittedly, this amount is not much, but it is a bonus that supplements the kcals lost directly through exercise.

Eat More, Weigh Less

Results of animal and human studies during the past 35 years have been equivocal and confusing regarding the effect of exercise on appetite and food intake. The data have shown that exercise decreases, increases, or has no effect upon food intake. Most studies have indicated that people either continued to eat the same amount or increased their food intake when they began exercising and were allowed to eat freely.

In an investigation of the effect of a year of jogging on previously sedentary middle-aged males, the subjects were encouraged not to reduce their food intake or to attempt to lose weight during the course of the study.[14] At the end of one year, the men who ran the most miles had lost the most fat. The more miles they ran, the more they increased their food intake. Those who jogged the most miles (up to 25 miles per week) lost the most fat and the most weight and had the greatest increase in food intake. Many studies have shown that active people consume more kcals, yet are leaner than inactive people.

Two studies at St. Luke's Hospital in New York showed that the effect of exercise on the appetite is regulated to some extent by how obese the person is at the start of the program.[15] After 57 days of moderate treadmill exercise, the obese female subjects had lost an average of 15 pounds. The women's caloric intake during exercise compared to the pre-exercise period was essentially unchanged. This study was repeated with women who were close to ideal weight according to insurance company charts. Moderate treadmill exercise produced an immediate surge in appetite, and the women maintained their "ideal body weight."

Exercise Stimulates Metabolism

Approximately 60% to 75% of the energy liberated from food is expended to maintain the essential functions of the body.[16] The energy to accomplish these functions is the **basal metabolic rate (BMR)** — the minimum amount of energy that the body expends to sustain life while at complete rest. The BMR is measured at least 12 hours since the last meal, after 8 hours of sleep, and in a thermally neutral environment (at a comfortable room temperature). Because these conditions are difficult to satisfy, they often are approximated, so that the BMR is estimated by the **resting metabolic rate (RMR)**. The RMR requires that measurements be taken 3 to 4 hours after the last meal, following a 30-minute rest period, in a thermally comfortable environment, on a day in which the person has not participated in vigorous physical activity.

Because of less muscle and more fat, the RMR of females is 5 to 10% lower than males and 15% lower than that of very muscular males. Males who are overweight primarily because of heavy musculature have higher RMRs and respond more readily to exercise/diet approaches to weight loss than overweight men whose excess weight is primarily fat.[17] The energy needed to sustain the RMR constitutes a significant amount of the total number of daily calories expended by the average adult. Then, from a weight-management perspective, it is advantageous to preserve or enhance the RMR and to do nothing to reduce it. Exercise fits the bill very nicely.

A persistent misconception regarding exercise is that it does not burn enough calories to make the effort worthwhile. Actually, consistent participation in aerobic exercise (such as walking, jogging, cycling, rowing, aerobic dance) will burn substantial kcals. Anaerobic activities such as weight training do not burn many kcals during the workout, but they build the muscle tissue that will require more kcals later on. Muscle-building activities are an investment in future weight control. In the long run, the increase in muscle mass increases metabolism so the body's kcal requirements increase even at rest. This is why activities for both cardiorespiratory development and muscular development are suggested for weight loss or weight maintenance or, for that matter, any well-rounded physical fitness program.

In the past, the decline in RMR was presumed to be a natural part of aging. But age per se has relatively little effect. The acquired changes accompanying aging are primarily responsible for the decline in RMR. Muscle tissue uses more oxygen and more calories than fat during rest or physical activity. Authorities estimate that we lose 3% to 5% of our active protoplasm (mostly muscle tissue) each decade after 25 years of age.[18] This loss is attributed directly to physical inactivity as we age and results in the all too common negative changes in body composition (amount of fat versus lean body tissue).

Physical activity is the key to weight management because it uses calories and accelerates metabolism. It also prevents or attenuates the weight-loss plateau that the majority of dieters experience. This plateau represents a period of time when weight loss decelerates substantially or stops temporarily.

For example, young and middle-aged individuals who were within plus or minus 5% of their ideal weight, as determined by height, weight, and frame size charts, illustrated the body composition changes that occur with age and physical inactivity.[19] Although both groups were within the ideal range for weight, the middle-aged subjects had twice as much body fat as the young subjects. These data show quite well that lost muscle weight that is replaced by a gain in fat weight produces negative changes in body composition even in the absence of weight gain. Fat is less dense than muscle, so it occupies more room in the body; hence, the change in the configuration of the body. Table 7.9 illustrates some of the changes in body composition that occur as we age. The examples are hypothetical, but they are based upon facts that have been generated over many years of research.

Subject 1 typifies the inactive person who maintains his body weight while aging but undergoes a change in body composition. His bathroom scales provide no clues regarding the change, but the mirror and the fit of his clothes do. This man must hold a tight rein on his appetite because his resting caloric requirements have diminished.

Subject 2 is inactive and chooses to lose weight with age to keep from becoming fatter — rare in U. S. society. He loses one quarter to one half a pound per year after age 30. This individual had lost muscle tissue and has reduced his body weight. His body composition has changed as a result; he is smaller all over. Because of the decline in metabolism from the loss of muscle, along with a lower body weight,

Table 7.9 Effects of Physical Inactivity on Body Composition

Subject	Body Weight at Age 20 (lbs)	Body Weight at Age 60 (lbs)	Activity Level	Lean Tissue*	Body Fat	Composition
1	150	150	Inactive	Lost 12%–20%	Gain	Changed
2	150	135	Inactive	Lost 12%–20%	No gain	Changed
3	150	165	Inactive	Lost 12%–20%	Gain	Changed
4	150	150	Active	No Loss	No gain	Unchanged

*The lean tissue values in the table apply to males. The same trend is evident to a lesser extent in females because women have less lean tissue to lose.

Source: Adapted from *Nutrition for Fitness and Sport*, by M. Williams (Dubuque, IA: Wm. C. Brown, 1992).

which diminishes the caloric cost of any weight-bearing movement, this individual must eat progressively less as the years pass to prevent a gain in fat tissue. Hunger would be a constant companion with this strategy.

Subject 3 probably is most representative of the typical American, who gains both fat and total weight with age. Subject 4 is physically active throughout life. He has little muscle loss and no gain in fat weight. Many examples of this modern-day phenomenon continue to jog, cycle, swim, and so on. Programs that build and maintain muscle tissue preserve the RMR and perpetuate a youthful body composition.

The Effect of Diet On Weight Control

Weight loss attempts in the United States have emphasized dietary restriction with continued sedentary living.[20] This combination has led to consistent failure. Weight loss with this method is temporary, and most of these weight watchers lose and gain weight many times during their life. The eating patterns established during the diet period are short-lived.

People in the United States have been, and continue to be, obsessed with losing weight. At any given time, about 40% of women and 25% of men are attempting to lose weight for reasons of physical appearance or health.[21] Unfortunately, 90% to 95% of all dieters regain all or most of the weight that they lost within five years.[22] Eat-less approaches to weight loss and permanent weight control have not worked and probably never will. Inexplicably, people continue to utilize weight-loss strategies that have failed them in the past. New attempts may feature new "diets," but calorie restriction remains the method of choice.

It is time to forget dieting as an effective weight-loss technique. The appropriate nutritional approach emphasizes sensible modifications in eating behavior that can be followed for a lifetime, not for just a few weeks or a few months. This means a nutritional approach that emphasizes a low-fat, high complex-carbohydrate style of eating. This, combined with sensible, progressive, and consistent exercise for a lifetime, should produce the permanent weight loss and control that people want.

Metabolism is affected adversely by calorie restriction.[23] In its quest for **homeostasis** (the tendency to maintain a constancy of internal conditions), the body adapts to the reduced-calorie intake by lowering the metabolic rate. This effort to economize in response to less food intake is a survival mechanism that protects people during lean times. Because the body learns to get by with less, the difference between calories eaten and the calories it needs narrows. This defense mechanism is what has made possible the survival of prisoners of war in concentration camps. Individuals who voluntarily reduce their food intake have the same result: a drop in RMR. As RMR decreases, so too does the effectiveness of dieting.

Regular vigorous exercise has the opposite effect: It accelerates the metabolic processes and increases body temperature during and after physical activity. The RMR might remain elevated for some time after exercise. Under exercise conditions, the body is spending kcals rather than hoarding them.

Metabolism represents the body's production of heat. Exercise increases heat production, oxygen demand, and calories used. Dieting without exercise, on the other hand, reduces metabolic heat production and, consequently, the number of calories burned. Some studies have shown that several weeks of a very low calorie diet (less than 800 kcals/day) resulted in a drop of heat production to 80% of the pre-diet level. This is counterproductive because weight loss under this procedure becomes more difficult. As the number of calories needed decreases, the difference between those needed and those consumed becomes smaller. The more restrictive the diet, the greater the loss of lean tissue and metabolic heat production.

Weight Cycling

Repeated weight loss and regain is referred to as **weight cycling** also known as cycle dieting and yo-yo dieting. Controversy has arisen regarding the health implications of weight cycling. Some evidence suggests that this practice, if it goes on a number of years, might increase the probability of developing cardiovascular disease. Others say a benefit might be associated with weight cycling: When people are in the weight-loss phase of the cycle, their blood pressure and blood fats decrease, along with their risk for Type II diabetes. In short, they are healthier during these periods of lighter body weight. When they regain weight, however, the risks return to pre-diet levels.[24] The surest course of action for overweight and obese people is to lose the weight and keep it off. Figure 7.4 shows the effects of frequent dieting without exercise on body weight.

Waist/Hip Ratio (WHR)

Obesity increases the risk of premature **morbidity** (the sick rate in a population) and **mortality** (the death rate in a population). The distribution of fat is as important as the amount of fat that is deposited. Fat that is distributed regionally in the abdomen, back, and chest — the male pattern, **android obesity** — increases the risk of heart attack, stroke, Type II diabetes, and some forms of cancer.[25] As few as 10 to 15 pounds stored in this manner increases the risk. Fat stored in the hips, buttocks, and thighs — the female pattern, or **gynoid obesity** — is not as risky, but it carries a higher risk than that associated with a normal body weight.

The pattern of fat deposition can be determined by calculating the waist/hip ratio (WHR). Ideally, the hips should be larger than the waist. Use a flexible tape to measure the circumference of your waist at the height of the navel. Then measure your hips at their largest circumference

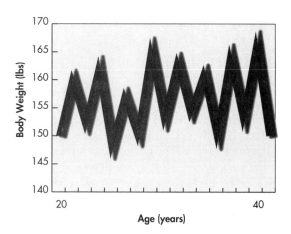

Figure 7.4 Effects of frequent dieting without exercise on body weight.

and divide the waist measurement by the hip measurement. The value obtained can be interpreted as follows:

◆ Females: If the WHR is .8 or greater, the risk is higher than normal

◆ Males: If the WHR is 1.0 or greater, the risk is higher than normal

Although the waist/hip ratio is a useful tool, an expert panel convened by the National Heart, Lung, and Blood Institute in 1998 concluded that a waist-circumference measurement alone was equally as good or better.[26] The risk for heart disease increases substantially when the waist circumference equals or exceeds 40 inches for males and 35 inches for females. The predictive power of waist circumference is unaffected by height, and its predictive power increases when combined with a body mass index (BMI) greater then 25 Kg/m². Body mass index is discussed later in this chapter.

Zuti and Golding investigated the relationship between exercise, diet, and weight loss,[27] analyzing the effects of three different strategies upon the quantity and quality of weight loss. Each strategy was designed to elicit a loss of 1 pound per week. The subjects were overweight women 25 to 45 years of age. A summary of the results of the study appears in Table 7.10.

The diet-only group reduced food intake by 500 kcals per day and did not exercise. The exercise-only group did not diet but increased physical activity by 500 kcals per day. The diet-and-exercise group reduced caloric intake by 250 kcals per day while increasing caloric expenditure by the same amount. The aim of all three strategies was to lose one pound per week (500 kcals × 7 days = 3500 kcals), and all three groups essentially accomplished this objective. The significant outcome of this study, however, was that 21% of the total weight loss in the diet-only group was in the form of lean tissue. This occurred despite a nutritionally sound diet of modest calorie restriction. The other two groups lost fat (the true goal of weight-loss programs) and gained rather than lost lean tissue.

Several other investigators have corroborated the results of this study, and all of them indicated that lean tissue is lost when diet restriction is not accompanied by exercise. The studies reinforced the need for including both sensible exercise and dietary modifications in a weight-loss program. The integrity of the muscular system can be protected only by participating in regular and systematic exercise, and this benefit occurs regardless of whether the person is dieting.

Some obese people seem to be diet-resistant; their weight remains stable even when they are following a low-calorie diet. This irony has been blamed variously upon an underactive thyroid, slow metabolism, or a hereditary tendency toward obesity. A number of studies have shown that the actual reason, in the majority of these cases, is that the subjects tended to underreport

Table 7.10 Summary of Zuti/Golding Study

Weight Loss Strategy	Fat Tissue Loss (lb)	Lean Tissue Loss (lb)	Total Weight Loss (lb)
Diet only	−9.3	−2.4	−11.7
Exercise only	−12.6	+2.0	−10.6
Diet and exercise	−13.0	+1.0	−12.0

Source: "Comparing Diet and Exercise as Weight-Reduction Tools," by B Zuti and L. Golding, *Physician and Sportsmedicine*, 4 (1976), 49.

their caloric intake and overestimate their physical activity. This dilemma was examined in a well-controlled study.[28] The researchers found that their diet-resistant subjects underestimated their food intake by 47% and overestimated their physical activity by 51%. The subjects perceived that their obesity was caused by genetic and metabolic factors rather than errors of judgment regarding caloric consumption and energy expenditure.

The American College of Sports Medicine (ACSM) produced a position paper in 1983, providing sensible guidelines. With some minor modifications (as identified by statements in brackets below) these are still appropriate today. Some of the important concepts addressed by ACSM are the following:[29]

1. A diet should provide at least 1200 kcals/day to increase the likelihood of obtaining the necessary nutrients to maintain good health. Diets that are calorically more restrictive are undesirable and potentially dangerous.

2. Food choices should be nutritionally balanced, palatable, and acceptable to the dieter.

3. Weight-loss goals should be moderate — no more than 2 pounds lost per week. [Today some experts support limiting weight loss to 1½ pounds per week.]

4. Behavior-modification techniques should be employed in conjunction with dietary modification and exercise to form a well-rounded approach to weight reduction.

5. An endurance-type exercise program is a must. The minimum amount of exercise recommended for weight loss includes participation 20 to 30 minutes per day, 3 times per week, at 60% of maximum heart rate. [If you expend 300 kcals per exercise session, you can exercise 3 times per week].

6. A resistance exercise program [primarily weight training] should accompany the walking or jogging program because it builds the muscle tissue that requires more calories than other bodily tissues, even during rest. The more muscle tissue, the higher is the metabolic rate of burning energy.

7. The dietary modifications and exercise program should be sustainable for a lifetime.

WEIGHT GAIN FOR UNDERWEIGHT PEOPLE

The focus thus far has been on weight loss rather than weight gain. Nevertheless, the purposeful gain of weight represents a real problem for people who are underweight. What constitutes underweight? This question has not been satisfactorily answered. In any case, actuarial statistics indicate that those who are significantly below the average in body weight have a higher expected mortality rate. Marked underweight can indicate underlying disease and is as much of a risk as obesity for early death.

Being underweight sometimes poses as much of a cosmetic problem for the individual as obesity does for an obese individual. An effective weight-gain program should include regular participation in resistance exercise, in conjunction with three well-balanced meals plus a couple of nutritious snacks between meals. Some commercial drinks are useful for increasing caloric consumption. Protein supplementation is unnecessary, though, and can be harmful in excess.

Despite herculean efforts, many underweight people find that gaining a pound is more difficult than losing a pound for the obese.

The amount and type of weight gain should be monitored closely. Gaining muscle tissue without increasing fat stores is desirable. Overeating without exercising will not accomplish this objective, nor will it enhance physical appearance. Body fat should not be increased unless the affected individuals are so thin that they are in danger of dipping into essential fat, which is necessary for the life processes.

MEASURING OVERWEIGHT

Overweight is defined as excess weight for one's height. It is assessed by using a height/weight chart or body mass index (BMI). If your weight falls above the acceptable range, you are overweight. This approach does not make allowances for body composition. It just provides information about weight status without taking into account the person's fluid, fat, or muscle make-up. Two people of the same sex, same height, and same weight conceivably could differ considerably in physical appearance because one may be carrying excess fat while the other is carrying substantial muscle tissue. Besides the difference in physical appearance, the risk of developing premature chronic disease is associated with excess fat, not muscle.

Body Mass Index (BMI)

A method for assessing overweight that is popular with medical and nutrition researchers is the body mass index (BMI). Some authorities consider it to be the best available method for assessing **percent body fat**.[30] Its inherent limitation — because it is based on height and weight — is similar to that of the height/weight tables. Muscular people can fall into the overweight category without being overfat. Advantages of this method are:

— the ease with which it can be determined

— the establishment of BMI categories that identify weight status

— the identification of BMI levels that constitute a risk for cardiovascular disease.

Body mass index can easily be determined from Table 7.11 by reading the directions at the top of the table. If your weight falls between two columns, however, you will have to extrapolate. For example, a person who is 68 inches tall and weighs 163 pounds is half the distance between 158 lbs and 164 pounds, which translates into half the distance between 24 and 25 Kg/M^2, or 24.5 KgM^2.

Interpretation of BMI is as follows:[31]

1. A BMI lower than 25 Kg/M^2 is acceptable.
2. A BMI of 25 to 29.9 Kg/M^2 is overweight.
3. A BMI equal to or greater than 30 Kg/M^2 is obese.

MEASURING BODY COMPOSITION

Body composition assessment requires the separation and quantification of lean tissue from fat. Many indirect methods for measuring this component have been developed but we will focus on just one — **skinfold** measurements.

Lean tissue includes all tissue except fat: muscle, bones, organs, fluid, and so on. Fat includes both essential and storage fat. **Essential fat**, found in the bone marrow, organs, muscles, intestines, and central nervous system, is indispensable to normal physiological functioning.

The amount of essential fat in the male body is equal to approximately 3% to 5% of the total body weight. The amount of essential fat in the female body is equal to about 11% to 14% of the total body weight. The disparity in the amount of essential fat between the sexes is probably because of sex-specific essential fat stored in a female's breasts, pelvic area, and thighs. Essential

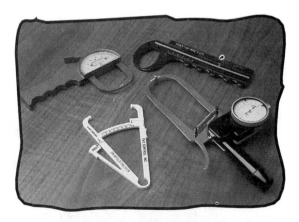

Various types of calipers
used to assess skinfold thickness.

fat constitutes a lower limit beyond which fat loss is undesirable and unhealthy because of the possibility of impaired normal physiological and biological functioning from such loss.

Storage fat is found in **adipose** (fat) tissue. For most people, this represents a substantial energy reserve. Adipose cells are found subcutaneously (under the skin) and around the organs, where they act as a buffer against physical trauma. Reducing excess storage fat is desirable for health and aesthetic reasons. Reasonable goals for total body fat (essential plus storage fat) differ by sex. Excellent values for males and females are 12% and 20%, respectively. Males are **overfat** when 25% or more of their weight is in the form of fat. Females are overfat when 32% or more of their weight is in the form of fat.

Skinfold measurement has become more commonplace ever since several low-cost calipers have made their way into the marketplace. In

Table 7.11 Body Mass Index Table BMI (kg/m²)

Directions: Each entry gives the body weight in pounds for a person of a given height and BMI. Pounds have been rounded to the nearest whole number. Find your height in the far left column and move horizontally across the row to your body weight. The number at the top of the column is your BMI.

Height (Inches)	19	20	21	22	23	24	25	26	27	28	29	30	35	40
						Body Weight (Pounds)								
58	91	96	100	105	110	115	119	124	129	134	138	143	167	191
59	94	99	104	109	114	119	124	128	133	138	143	148	173	198
60	97	102	107	112	118	123	128	133	138	143	148	153	179	204
61	100	106	111	116	122	127	132	137	143	148	153	158	185	211
62	104	109	115	120	126	131	136	142	147	153	158	164	191	218
63	107	113	118	124	130	135	141	146	152	158	163	169	197	225
64	110	116	122	128	134	140	145	151	157	163	169	174	204	232
65	114	120	126	132	138	144	150	156	162	168	174	180	210	240
66	118	124	130	136	142	148	155	161	167	173	179	186	216	247
67	121	127	134	140	146	153	159	166	172	178	185	191	223	255
68	125	131	138	144	151	158	164	171	177	184	190	197	230	262
69	128	135	142	149	155	162	169	176	182	189	196	203	236	270
70	132	139	146	153	160	167	174	181	188	195	202	207	243	278
71	136	143	150	157	165	172	179	186	193	200	208	215	230	286
72	140	147	154	162	169	177	184	191	199	296	213	221	258	294
73	144	151	159	166	174	182	189	197	204	212	219	227	265	302
74	148	155	163	171	179	186	194	202	210	218	225	233	272	311
75	152	160	168	176	184	192	200	208	216	224	232	240	279	319
76	156	164	172	180	189	197	205	213	221	230	238	246	287	328

skilled hands, some of them correlate quite well (.90) with the more expensive brands found in most exercise physiology labs.

The rationale for the skinfold technique is that approximately half of the body's fat is located directly beneath the skin. Therefore, the skinfold — which consists of a double layer of skin and the underlying fat — can be measured with a caliper. Tables for age and sex are used to convert skinfold measurement (in millimeters) to percent fat. These are given in Tables 7.12 and 7.13.

To become proficient, the person administering the skinfold test practices measuring the different sites for all ages and both sexes. The method can be standardized by observing the following suggestions:

1. Mark each site according to the directions given in Figure 7.5.

2. Take two measurements at each site, unless the two differ by more than 1 millimeter. In that case, take a third measurement and average the two closest readings.

3. Apply the calipers about ¼ inch to ½ inch below the fingers. This allows the calipers rather than the fingers to compress the skinfold.

4. Ensure that the calipers maintain contact with the skinfold for 2 to 5 seconds so the reading can stabilize.

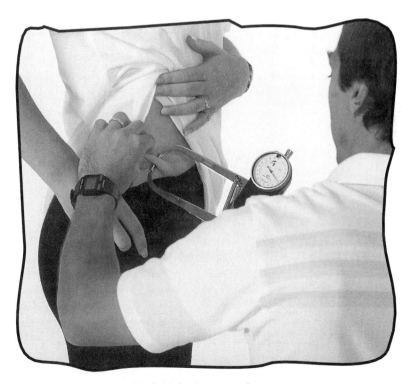

Skinfold thickness technique
for determining body composition.

Table 7.12   Percent Fat Estimates For Men*

Sum of Skinfolds (mm)	Under 22	23 to 27	28 to 32	33 to 37	38 to 42	43 to 47	48 to 52	53 to 57	Over 57
					Age to the Last Year				
8– 10	1.3	1.8	2.3	2.9	3.4	3.9	4.5	5.0	5.5
11– 13	2.2	2.8	3.3	3.9	4.4	4.9	5.5	6.0	6.5
14– 16	3.2	3.8	4.3	4.8	5.4	5.9	6.4	7.0	7.5
17– 19	4.2	4.7	5.3	5.8	6.3	6.9	7.4	8.0	8.5
20– 22	5.1	5.7	6.2	6.8	7.3	7.9	8.4	8.9	9.5
23– 25	6.1	6.6	7.2	7.7	8.3	8.8	9.4	9.9	10.5
26– 28	7.0	7.6	8.1	8.7	9.2	9.8	10.3	10.9	11.4
29– 31	8.0	8.5	9.1	9.6	10.2	10.7	11.3	11.8	12.4
32– 34	8.9	9.4	10.0	10.5	11.5	11.6	12.2	12.8	13.3
35– 37	9.8	10.4	10.9	11.5	12.0	12.6	13.1	13.7	14.3
38– 40	10.7	11.3	11.8	12.4	12.9	13.5	14.1	14.6	15.2
41– 43	11.6	12.2	12.7	13.3	13.8	14.4	15.0	15.5	16.1
44– 46	12.5	13.1	13.6	14.2	14.7	15.3	15.9	16.4	17.0
47– 49	13.4	13.9	14.5	15.1	15.6	16.2	16.8	17.3	17.9
50– 52	14.3	14.8	15.4	15.9	16.5	17.1	17.6	18.2	18.8
53– 55	15.1	15.7	16.2	16.8	17.4	17.9	18.5	19.1	19.7
56– 58	16.0	16.5	17.1	17.7	18.2	18.8	19.4	20.0	20.5
59– 61	16.9	17.4	17.9	18.5	19.1	19.7	20.2	20.8	21.4
62– 64	17.6	18.2	18.8	19.4	19.9	20.5	21.1	21.7	22.2
65– 67	18.5	19.0	19.6	20.2	20.8	21.3	21.9	22.5	23.1
68– 70	19.3	19.9	20.4	21.0	21.6	22.2	22.7	23.3	23.9
71– 73	20.1	20.7	21.2	21.8	22.4	23.0	23.6	24.1	24.7
74– 76	20.9	21.5	22.0	22.6	23.2	23.8	24.4	25.0	25.5
77– 79	21.7	22.2	22.8	23.4	24.0	24.6	25.2	25.8	26.3
80– 82	22.4	23.0	23.6	24.2	24.8	25.4	25.9	26.5	27.1
83– 85	23.2	23.8	24.4	25.0	25.5	26.1	26.7	27.3	27.9
86– 88	24.0	24.5	25.1	25.7	26.3	26.9	27.5	28.1	28.7
89– 91	24.7	25.3	25.9	26.5	27.1	27.6	28.2	28.8	29.4
92– 94	25.4	26.0	26.6	27.2	27.8	28.4	29.0	29.6	30.2
95– 97	26.1	26.7	27.3	27.9	28.5	29.1	29.7	30.3	30.9
98–100	26.9	27.4	28.0	28.6	29.2	29.8	30.4	31.0	31.6
101–103	27.5	28.1	28.7	29.3	29.9	30.5	31.1	31.7	32.3
104–106	28.2	28.8	29.4	30.0	30.6	31.2	31.8	32.4	33.0
107–109	28.9	29.5	30.1	30.7	31.3	31.9	32.5	33.1	33.7
110–112	29.6	30.2	30.8	31.4	32.0	32.6	33.2	33.8	34.4
113–115	30.2	30.8	31.4	32.0	32.6	33.2	33.8	34.5	35.1
116–118	30.9	31.5	32.1	32.7	33.3	33.9	34.5	35.1	35.7
119–121	31.5	32.1	32.7	33.3	33.9	34.5	35.1	35.7	36.4
122–124	32.1	32.7	33.3	33.9	34.5	35.1	35.8	36.4	37.0
125–127	32.7	33.3	33.9	34.5	35.1	35.8	36.4	37.0	37.6

*Sum of chest, abdominal, and thigh skinfolds.

"Practical Assessment of Body Composition," by A. S. Jackson and M. L. Pollock, *The Physician and Sportsmedicine*, 13:5 (1985) 76–90. Reprinted by permission.

Table 7.13 Percent Fat Estimates For Women*

Sum of Skinfolds (mm)	Under 22	23 to 27	28 to 32	33 to 37	38 to 42	43 to 47	48 to 52	53 to 57	Over 57
				Age to the Last Year					
23– 25	9.7	9.9	10.2	10.4	10.7	10.9	11.2	11.4	11.7
26– 28	11.0	11.2	11.5	11.7	12.0	12.3	12.5	12.7	13.0
29– 31	12.3	12.5	12.8	13.0	13.3	13.5	13.8	14.0	14.3
32– 34	13.6	13.8	14.0	14.3	14.5	14.8	15.0	15.3	15.5
35– 37	14.8	15.0	15.3	15.5	15.8	16.0	16.3	16.5	16.8
38– 40	16.0	16.3	16.5	16.7	17.0	17.2	17.5	17.7	18.0
41– 43	17.2	17.4	17.7	17.9	18.2	18.4	18.7	18.9	19.2
44– 46	18.3	18.6	18.8	19.1	19.3	19.6	19.8	20.1	20.3
47– 49	19.5	19.7	20.0	20.2	20.5	20.7	21.0	21.2	21.5
50– 52	20.6	20.8	21.1	21.3	21.6	21.8	22.1	22.3	22.6
53– 55	21.7	21.9	22.1	22.4	22.6	22.9	23.1	23.4	23.6
56– 58	22.7	23.0	23.2	23.4	23.7	23.9	24.2	24.4	24.7
59– 61	23.7	24.0	24.2	24.5	24.7	25.0	25.2	25.5	25.7
62– 64	24.7	25.0	25.2	25.5	25.7	26.0	26.2	26.4	26.7
65– 67	25.7	25.9	26.2	26.4	26.7	26.9	27.2	27.4	27.7
68– 70	26.6	26.9	27.1	27.4	27.6	27.9	28.1	28.4	28.6
71– 73	27.5	27.8	28.0	28.3	28.5	28.8	29.0	29.3	29.5
74– 76	28.4	28.8	28.9	29.2	29.4	29.7	29.9	30.2	30.4
77– 79	29.3	29.5	29.8	30.0	30.3	30.5	30.8	31.0	31.3
80– 82	30.1	30.4	30.6	30.9	31.1	31.4	31.6	31.9	32.1
83– 85	30.9	31.2	31.4	31.7	31.9	32.2	32.4	32.7	32.9
86– 88	31.7	32.0	32.2	32.5	32.7	32.9	33.2	33.4	33.7
89– 91	32.5	32.7	33.0	33.2	33.5	33.7	33.9	34.2	34.4
92– 94	33.2	33.4	33.7	33.9	34.2	34.4	34.7	34.9	35.2
95– 97	33.9	34.1	34.4	34.6	34.9	35.1	35.4	35.6	35.9
98–100	34.6	34.8	35.1	35.3	35.5	35.8	36.0	36.3	36.5
101–103	35.3	35.4	35.7	35.9	36.2	36.4	36.7	36.9	37.2
104–106	35.8	36.1	36.3	36.6	36.8	37.1	37.3	37.5	37.8
107–109	36.4	36.7	36.9	37.1	37.4	37.6	37.9	38.1	38.4
110–112	37.0	37.2	37.5	37.7	38.0	38.2	38.5	38.7	38.9
113–115	37.5	37.8	38.0	38.2	38.5	38.7	39.0	39.2	39.5
116–118	38.0	38.3	38.5	38.8	39.0	39.3	39.5	39.7	40.0
119–121	38.5	38.7	39.0	39.2	39.5	39.7	40.0	40.2	40.5
122–124	39.0	39.2	39.4	39.7	39.9	40.2	40.4	40.7	40.9
125–127	39.4	39.6	39.9	40.0	40.4	40.6	40.9	41.1	41.4
128–130	39.8	40.0	40.3	40.5	40.8	41.0	41.3	41.5	41.8

*Sum of triceps, suprailium, and thigh skinfolds..

"Practical Assessment of Body Composition," by A. S. Jackson and M. L. Pollock, *The Physician and Sportsmedicine*, 13:5 (1985) 76–90. Reprinted by permission.

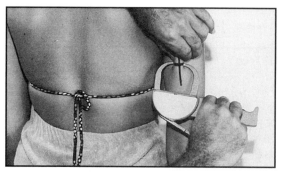

Triceps Skinfold. Take a vertical fold on the midline of the upper arm over the triceps halfway between the acromion and olecranon processes (tip of shoulder to tip of elbow). The arm should be extended and relaxed when the measurement is taken.

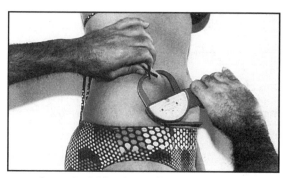

Suprailium Skinfold. Take a diagonal fold above the crest of the ilium directly below the mid-axilla (armpit).

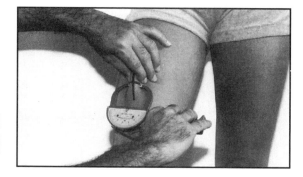

Thigh Skinfold. Take a vertical fold on the front of the thigh midway between the hip and knee joint.

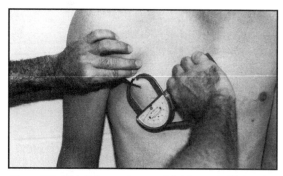

Chest Skinfold. Take a diagonal fold one-half the distance between the anterior axillary line and nipple.

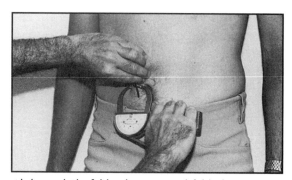

Abdominal Skinfold. Take a vertical fold about 3/8 inch from the navel.

Figure 7.5 Skinfold measurement sites.

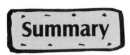

Summary

- Metabolism is the sum total of chemical reactions whereby the energy liberated from food is made available to the body. It consists of two processes — anabolism and catabolism.

- The Food Guide Pyramid has replaced the basic four food group.

- The food labels mandated by the federal government for processed food give quantities of various nutrients and caloric values that help consumers make more informed food choices.

- Carbohydrates consist of simple sugars and starches.

- Sugar causes tooth decay but is not an independent risk factor for chronic diseases except in rare cases.

- Sugar consumption continues to rise in the United States.

- Fiber is an indigestible polysaccharide that is beneficial to health. The two types of dietary fiber are soluble and insoluble.

- Carbohydrates yield 4 kcals/gram.

- Fats are energy-dense, yielding 9 kcals/gram.

- Saturated fats come from animal flesh, dairy products, and tropical oils. This type of fat raises serum cholesterol levels.

- Unsaturated fats come from plants and should constitute the majority of the fat we consume.

- Dietary fat should be less than 30% of the total caloric intake.

- Transfatty acids could be as harmful as saturated fats. This artificial fat (made through the process of hydrogenation) makes up 5% to 10% of the fat in the average U.S. diet.

- Protein intake should be about 12% of the total calories consumed.

- Adults need .8 of a gram of protein per kg of body weight; endurance athletes require about twice this amount.

- The fat-soluble vitamins are A, D, E, and K; the water-soluble vitamins are C and B complex.

- Antioxidant vitamins are thought to play an important role in preventing cardiovascular disease and cancer.

- Free radicals are harmful body products that damage cells; they can be contained by consuming abundance of antioxidant vitamins, found in vegetables and fruits.

- Minerals are inorganic substances that exist freely in nature and the body requires them as major minerals or trace minerals.

- Exercise is an important component of weight management because it burns calories and stimulates metabolism. Dieters decrease their caloric intake but, without exercise, reduce their metabolism and lean body tissue instead of fat.

- Most dieters regain the lost weight within 5 years.

- Weight cycling (yo-yo dieting) increases the risk of cardiovascular disease.

- Android obesity (male) increases the risk of heart attack, stroke, Type II diabetes, and some forms of cancer. Gynoid obesity (female) likewise increases the risk for "lifestyle diseases."

- Body mass index (BMI) is a good method for determining one's weight status.

- Males have less essential fat than females.

- Skinfold measurement techniques are inexpensive, quick, and effective for measuring percent body fat.

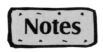

1. S. Margen and the Editors, "Wellness Nutrition Counter," *University of California at Berkeley Wellness Letter* (NY: Rebus, 1997).

2 B. Liebman, "Sugar: The Sweetening of the American Diet," *Nutrition Action Health Letter*, 25:9 (Nov. 1998), 1–7.

3. M. Jacobson, "Liquid Candy," *Nutrition Action Health Letter*, 25:9 (Nov. 1998), 8.

4. "Myth: Fruit Juice Concentration Is a More Healthful Sweetener Than Sugar," *University of California at Berkeley Wellness Letter*, 9:2 (Sept. 1993), 8.

5. L.J. Dahl, "Sugars and Fats: The Tip of the Food Pyramid," *Cardi Sense*, 4:2 (1994), 6.

6. "Mediterranean Diet: A Fish Connection," *Harvard Heart Letter*, 7:8 (April 1997), 1–2.

7. T. Byers, "Hardened Fats, Hardened Arteries?" *New England Journal of Medicine*, 337:21 (Nov. 20, 1997), 1554–1545.

8. "What to Make of Recent News that Butter is Better Than Margarine," *Environmental Nutrition*, 21:1 (Jan. 1998), 3.

9. S.N. Steen, and G. Butterfield, "Diet and Nutrition," *ACSM's Resource Manual for Guidelines for Exercise Testing and Prescription*, 3d ed., edited by J.L. Roitman (Baltimore: Williams and Wilkins, 1998).

10. B.N. Ames, M.K. Shigenaga, and T.M. Hagen, "Oxidants, Antioxidants, and the Degenerative Diseases of Aging," *Proceedings of the National Academy of Sciences*, 90 (1993) 7915–7922.

11. B. Liebman, "The Salt Shake Out," *Nutrition Action Health Letter*, 21:2 (March 1994), 1.

12. *ACSM's Resource Manual for Exercise Testing and Prescription.*

13. D.C. Nieman, *Exercise Testing and Prescription A Health Related Approach* (Mountain View, CA: Mayfield, 1999).

14. P.D. Wood, et al., "Increased Exercise Level and Plasma Lipoprotein Concentrations: A One-year Randomized, Controlled Study in Sedentary Middle-Aged Men," *Metabolism*, 32 (1983), 31.

15. P. Wood, *California Diet and Exercise Program* (Mountain View, CA: Anderson World Books, 1983).

16. Nieman.

17. C. Pierre, "Maximizing Metabolism: Can Calorie Burning Be Increased?" *Environmental Nutrition*, 12 (Feb. 1989), 1.

18. R.A. Robergs and S.O. Roberts, *Exercise Physiology* (St. Louis: Mosby, 1997).

19. M. Williams, *Nutrition for Fitness and Sport* (Dubuque, IA: Wm. C Brown, 1992).

20. "Losing Weight: A New Attitude Emerges," *Harvard Heart Letter*, 4:7 (March 1994), 1.

21. "Heavy News," *University of California at Berkeley Wellness Letter*, 10:5 (Feb. 1994), 2.

22. S. Margolis and L.J. Cheskin, *Weight Control*, (New York: Medletter Associates, 1998).

23. Nieman.

24. "Yo-Yo Diets Aren't Risky, After All," *Health*, 9:1 (1995), 18.

25. J.P. Despres, "Viceral Obesity, Insulin Resistance, and Dyslipidemia: Contribution of Endurance Exercise Training to the Treatment of Plurimetabolic Syndrome," *Exercise and Sport Sciences Reviews*, 25 (1997), 271–300.

26. NHLBI Obesity Education Initiative Expert Panel, *Clinical Guidelines on the Identification, Evaluation and Treatment of Overweight and Obesity in Adults* (Washington, DC: National Heart, Lung, and Blood Institute, 1998).

27. B. Zuti and L. Golding, "Comparing Diet and Exercise as Weight Reduction Tools," *Physician and Sportsmedicine*, 4 (1976), 49.

28. S.W. Lichtman et al., "Discrepancy Between Self-Reported and Actual Caloric Intake and Exercise in Obese Subjects," *New England Journal of Medicine*, 327 (1992), 1893.

29. American College of Sports Medicine. "Proper and Improper Weight Loss Programs," *Medicine and Science in Sports and Exercise*, 15 (1983), ix.

30. *ACSM's Guidelines for Exercise Testing and Prescription.*

31. "Guidelines Call More Americans Overweight," *Harvard Health Letter*, 23:10 (Aug. 1998), 7.

Prevention and Treatment of Walking and Jogging Injuries

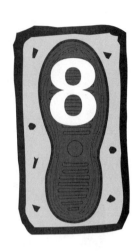

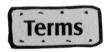
Terms

Amenorrhea
Concentric muscle contraction
Eccentric muscle contraction
Estrogen
Inflammation
Orthotic
RICE principle

Exercise participants will incur an injury or two if they exercise long enough. Fortunately, most injuries are minor and respond to minimal levels of treatment. The aim of this chapter is to reinforce the importance of preventing injuries and to acquaint you with recognizable symptoms and effective treatments for some common injuries. Recognizing the symptoms is the first step in treating the injury, and treatment should begin as soon as possible after incurring an injury.

PRINCIPLES OF INJURY PREVENTION

The often-heard adage, "an ounce of prevention is worth a pound of cure," is applicable when embarking upon a walking or jogging program. It continues to be sound advice even for seasoned participants, because after an injury-free period, some people become complacent and disregard the principles that contributed to their lack of injury. The best way to deal with injuries is to prevent them in the first place. Previous chapters focused upon the principles of training designed to promote aerobic fitness with maximum safety. These include the following:

1. Contain your enthusiasm. Enthusiasm is necessary for success, but too much can lead to overexertion and injury. You should increase the distance or decrease the time required to cover a given distance slowly and progressively.

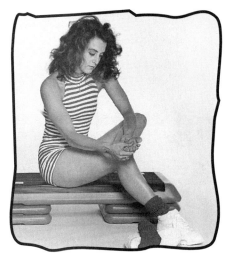

Recognize the signs of an injury
and treat it immediately.

2. If you have risk factors or are older than 45 years of age, obtain clearance for jogging by a physician.

3. Individualize your program to meet your aims and objectives.

4. Do not exceed 85% of maximal heart rate for the exercise intensity of each workout.

5. In the early stages of the program, keep the duration of each workout within the 20- to 30-minute range, and lengthen it as fitness improves.

6. In the beginning, walk or jog every other day and increase the frequency to a level that is consistent with physical improvement and the program objectives.

7. Wear quality walking or jogging shoes.

8. Adjust the intensity and duration of the workout according to the environmental conditions.

9. Hydrate fully prior to the workout, and continue to drink liquids during and after the workout.

10. Follow sound warm-up and cool-down procedures.

11. Work to improve your walking and jogging form.

12. Choose surfaces that are less likely to promote injuries.

TREATING COMMON INJURIES

In treating injuries, a general formula is provided by RICE. Common specific injuries are those to the hamstring and achilles tendon, blisters and chafing, and back pain.

General Treatment: The RICE Principle

The **RICE** (rest, ice, compression, elevation) formula will help to reduce pain, swelling, and **inflammation**.[1]

1. *Rest:* Rest if movement produces pain in the affected area.

2. *Ice:* Apply ice immediately for 15 to 20 minutes, and repeat ice application every few hours. Do not apply ice for more than 20 minutes at a time. A convenient way to apply ice is to put crushed ice or ice cubes in a large plastic freezer bag and place it on the injured area. As the ice melts, it will not leak.

3. *Compression:* Use an elastic bandage to wrap the injured area between icing. Do not keep the wrap on when you sleep, and loosen it if the injured area begins to throb or change color.

4. *Elevation:* Raise the injured area to keep down the swelling. Do this several times during the day.

Treating Selected Injuries

The following injuries are the most common of injuries to walkers and joggers.

Achilles Tendon Injuries

The achilles tendon connects the calf muscle to the heel of the foot. Achilles tendonitis is a painful inflammation often accompanied by swelling. Jogging uphill, walking or jogging shoes with inflexible soles, and failing to maintain a

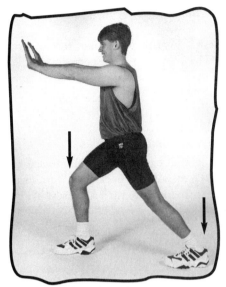

Exercise for prevention
and relief of achilles tendonitis.

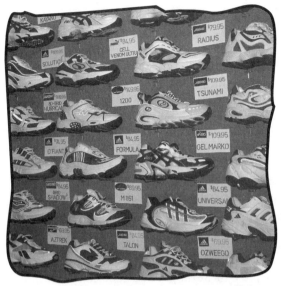

Properly fitting shoes are recommended
to prevent exercise-related injuries.

stretching program are the three most frequent causes of achilles tendonitis. Symptoms include burning pain, which usually appears early in the workout and then subsides until the exercise ends, at which time the pain reappears and progressively worsens.

Treatment includes icing the tendon followed by gently stretching. Prevention involves daily stretching to increase flexibility of the calf and the use of quality walking or jogging shoes.[2] Preventive maintenance is important because the tendon can tear or rupture under stress. In the latter case, surgery becomes the only effective treatment, but either situation leads to a long period of inactivity.[3]

Blisters

Blisters are painful friction burns of a minor nature that result in fluid-filled sacs of various sizes. Blisters can be prevented by wearing properly fitted shoes and clean socks and using the correct footstrike. In addition, foot or talcum powder may be sprinkled inside socks and shoes to reduce friction.

Moleskin (toughskin) can be applied to areas of the feet that tend to blister. "Hot spots"

are reddened areas that will become blisters quickly if preventive measures are not taken. If a blister forms:

1. Wash the area thoroughly with soap and water.

2. Apply a generous coat of iodine to the blister and the surrounding area.

3. With a sterile needle, puncture the blister at its base and squeeze out the accumulated fluid.

4. Apply an antiseptic medication and a sterile dressing.

5. Continue exercise after treatment by cutting a "doughnut" from foam rubber and taping it over the blister.

Chafing

Chafing occurs in areas that are subject to a lot of friction. For example, people with large thighs that rub together experience chafing. This a minor but aggravating injury that can be prevented easily by applying a generous coat of vaseline to susceptible areas prior to the workout. Treatment for chafing is to immediately cease walking and jogging with the onset of irritation, and to apply an antiseptic lotion.

Chondromalacia Patella

Chondromalacia patella (*chondro* = cartilage; *malacia* = softening; patella = kneecap) is commonly referred to as "runner's knee." This describes a condition in which the kneecap tracks laterally rather than vertically during flexion and extension of the leg. Typical symptoms are soreness around and under the kneecap, particularly when jogging uphill or climbing stairs. The pain must be eliminated before resuming jogging safely. Treatment includes resting, applying ice, and taking aspirin every 4 hours for several weeks. Ice treatment should be discontinued after 24 to 36 hours and replaced with moist heat application several times per day as long as needed.

When pain abates, the jogger can begin progressive resistance exercises to strengthen the quadriceps group (large muscles in the front of the thigh) and a low-intensity graduated jogging program. Preventive measures include:

1. Using orthotic devices (supports placed in jogging shoes to compensate for biomechanical problems); these are designed to prevent abnormal motions in the foot and lower leg during jogging

2. Avoiding hard running surfaces such as concrete sidewalks

3. Abstaining from sloped or hilly terrain

4. Keeping stair-climbing to a minimum.

Hamstring Injuries

The hamstrings are a group of muscles in the back of the thigh. The muscles in this group are subject to strains and tears. There is usually a specific area of pain directly over the area of injury. Muscles strains typically occur within the belly or central part of the muscle. Severe strains occur in the tendon where the muscle originates or connects to the bones. Hamstring tears occur either high in the thigh next to the buttocks or low just above the knee. When tears are on the inside of the thigh, they are usually close to the groin.

The RICE principle applies to hamstring injuries. The exerciser can perform mild static stretching of the hamstrings as long as this is not accompanied by pain. Forced stretches can aggravate the injury.

Low-Back Pain

Strains that cause the muscles to spasm constitute 90% of all low-back pain. Strains are attributed to many and varied causes. Those that commonly precipitate problems for walkers and joggers are:

1. Weak abdominal muscles,

2. Tight low-back and hamstring muscles

3. Overuse — increasing the mileage too rapidly

4. Faulty mechanics, particularly too much forward lean.

Preventive measures include daily stretching of the lower back and hamstrings, strengthening of the abdominals, slowly increasing the distance, and improving faulty walking and jogging mechanics. Walking and jogging strengthen the muscles of the lower back; stretching exercises keep them from shortening. At the same time, the abdominal muscles have to be strengthened because they provide some support to the spinal column in holding up the weight of the torso. Treatment of low-back pain includes rest, aspirin, and a firm mattress with a bedboard.

Morton's Neuroma

Morton's neuroma results in burning pain between the third and fourth toes, usually as a result of repetitive trauma such as that experienced by runners. Trauma is the primary cause, and pain is the primary symptom. Pain is the result of scar tissue (fibrosis) impinging upon the sensory digital nerve. It may be constant, or it might appear after walking or jogging on a hard surface. Narrow shoes, particularly high-heeled shoes, should be avoided.

Treatment includes the use of metatarsal bars or pads worn across the ball of the foot, shoes with a wide toebox, and local injection of a steroid preparation. Rest is suggested as long as the individual responds with pain to finger pressure at the site. If all of the above fail, surgery will be required. Prevention includes wearing walking, jogging, and everyday shoes that are roomy in the toebox, well padded under the balls of the feet, and flexible. Walking and jogging on softer surfaces also helps.

Muscle Cramps

Muscle cramps are sudden, powerful, involuntary muscle contractions that produce considerable pain. Some cramps recur — the muscles repeatedly contract and relax — and others produce steady, continuous contraction. Preventive measures include a gradual warm-up that includes stretching exercises. Overfatigue should be avoided.

Causes associated with muscle cramping are difficult to establish. Fatigue, depletion of body fluids and minerals, and loss of muscle coordination all have been implicated.

Muscle cramps should not be massaged because of possible underlying blood vessel damage and internal bleeding. Vigorous massage in this case would aggravate the condition and promote additional damage. Treatment includes applying firm, consistent pressure at the site of the cramp, followed by the application of ice and then stretching the affected muscle.

Muscle Soreness

Muscle soreness after walking and jogging is probably attributable to microscopic tears in muscle fibers and damage to muscle membranes. This damage is partially responsible for the localized pain, tenderness, and swelling that exercisers experience 24 to 48 hours after the workout. Downhill running and walking have been implicated in delayed muscle soreness. In downhill running, the leg muscles undergo **eccentric muscle contraction**. They produce force as they lengthen. Running uphill produces the opposite effect as the muscles undergo **concentric muscle contraction** to provide the lift needed to negotiate the upgrade.

To expand upon this concept, when a weight is lifted, the muscles contract concentrically to produce the force needed to raise the weight against the force of gravity. When the weight is returned to the starting position, the muscles contract eccentrically, lengthen, and produce the same amount of force to slow their descent. This portion of the movement is what results in delayed muscle soreness.

In a simple but ingenious study, the subjects exercised by consistently stepping onto a box with one leg and stepping down with the other. The step-up represented the concentric contraction, and the step-down the eccentric contraction. The subjects experienced pain, which peaked 48 hours after the exercise in the eccentrically exercised leg only.[4]

The delayed soreness experienced with eccentric exercise is probably attributable to the recruitment of only a few muscle fibers that must produce great tension to do the work. Untrained people have more delayed muscle soreness than trained people.

Delayed muscle soreness can be prevented by keeping the intensity, duration, and frequency of exercise within one's ability level, by progressing slowly, by doing daily stretching exercises, and by walking and jogging on a flat surface in the initial stages of training. As fitness improves, uphill and downhill walking and running are carefully included in the routine. Soreness is treated with rest as well as stretching the affected muscles several times per day.

Plantar Fasciitis

Occasionally, an exerciser experiences low-grade pain beneath the heel of one or both feet. In mild cases, the person feels this pain during jogging, but more severe cases produce pain upon walking also. The pain results from microscopic tears and inflammation of the connective tissue (planter fascia) beneath the heel. Treatment consists of cold therapy several times a day for the first few days, rest, anti-inflammatory drugs, heel pads, and possibly orthotic correction. **Orthotics** are supports placed in the walking and running shoes, designed to correct biomechanical problems. Prevention involves well-fitting, well-cushioned walking and jogging shoes and a stretching program that includes stretching the calf and achilles tendon.

Shin Splints

Shin splints produce pain that radiates along the inner surface of the large bone of the lower leg (see Figure 8.1). This condition is caused by running or walking on hard surfaces in improper shoes. It is most prevalent in unconditioned and novice exercisers who do too much too soon. Jogging or walking in one direction on a banked track or banked road shoulder can contribute to shin splints. Shin splints are the most common running injury.[5] Overweight/obesity can contribute to shin splints.

Pain associated with this injury manifests itself gradually. Initially it occurs after the workout, but as training continues, it tends to show up during the workout. In severe cases, pain accompanies walking and stair-climbing. Treatment includes rest, application of ice, wrapping or taping the shin, and placing heel lifts in the shoes.

The following exercises might help.

Toe Flexor

1. Sit in a chair with the bare feet approximately shoulder-width apart.

2. Place a towel on the floor in front of both feet, allowing the toes to overlap the near edge of the towel.

3. Repeatedly curl the toes to pull the towel toward you so it ends up under the arch of the feet.

The heels must be in contact with the floor at all times. You may place a weight, such as a book or a can of food on the towel to increase the resistance.

Toe Extensor   This is the reverse of the toe flexor exercise. By reversing the action of the toes, you will push the towel away from you and return it to the original position. Keep your heels on the floor.

Sandsweeper

1. Sit on a chair with one bare foot on the lateral edge of a towel.

2. Grasp the towel with the toes, and pivot on the heel to the right to sweep the towel in that direction.

3. Return the foot to the starting position and repeat until the towel has been moved completely to the right.

4. Replace the towel in the original position and sweep to the left.

5. Repeat with the other foot.

Shin splints are best prevented rather than treated. Preventive measures include wearing quality walking or jogging shoes, gradually adjust to the rigors of training, avoid hard surfaces and hilly terrain, use the proper heel-toe strike, and daily use the exercises described previously.

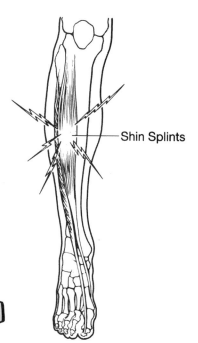

— Shin Splints

Figure 8.1

Shin splints.

Stress Fractures

Stress fractures are tiny, often microscopic breaks in bones. The bones of the feet and shins are particularly affected. Symptoms include one or all of the following: dull ache, local tenderness, and swelling. Pressure applied to the site of injury also produces pain.

This is a classic injury of overuse. Exercisers who are logging too many miles, exercising too often, and exercising on hard surfaces are candidates for stress fractures. Surfaces that have little or no "give" or "resiliency" force the body to absorb more of the shock.[6] This applies to joggers in particular because of the high shock of landing. Quality jogging shoes are a must, but they can absorb only a portion of the shock.

Women who are training heavily are susceptible to stress fractures, particularly if they become lean enough so their menstrual cycle stops, in which case the production of **estrogen** also stops (female sex hormone). Estrogen protects the bones from thinning out. A female runner who has had **amenorrhea** for a couple of years has lost a significant amount of bony tissue, and this, in combination with vigorous training, leaves her vulnerable to stress fractures. The risk of stress fractures for women can be reduced by cutting back on mileage and by not becoming so lean as to interrupt the menstrual cycle.

If a stress fracture has been diagnosed, rest is essential. The physician will advise when the person can return to physical activity. At that point, these people cannot pick up where they left off when they were injured. They should start at a low level and gradually increase the duration, frequency, and — lastl — the intensity of exercise. Stretching properly before and after exercise is essential, as are walking and jogging surfaces that have some "give." Preferred surfaces are artificial surfaces (such as those found on football fields and running tracks), flat, grassy surfaces free of holes (such as public parks and golf courses), and cinder running tracks. Motorized treadmills offer resilient surface for walking and jogging.

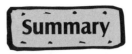

Summary

- Common-sense safety principles will help to prevent exercise-related injuries.
- The RICE principle is the general treatment suggested for many types of exercise-related injuries.
- Quality walking or jogging shoes are essential.
- The novice should start by walking or jogging every other day, then increasing the frequency to a level consistent with improvement and program objectives.
- Frequency and duration of exercise should be increased before increasing the intensity.
- The intensity and duration of the workout are adjusted to accommodate the environmental conditions.
- The exerciser should hydrate fully prior to working out and continue to drink liquid during and after exercising.
- Sound warm-up and cool-down procedures are part of a preventive program.
- Form is important in a walking or jogging program.
- Walking and jogging surfaces affect the risk of injury and should be selected carefully.
- Prevention of achilles tendon injuries includes daily stretching of the achilles tendon and calf muscles as well as wearing quality walking and jogging shoes. Treatment includes icing and daily stretching.
- Blisters may be prevented by wearing properly fitted shoes, clean socks, talcum powder sprinkled inside the shoes and socks, and by employing proper foot strike. Treatment involves puncturing the blister with a sterile needle so the fluid can be removed and the application of a strike bandage.
- Chafing can be prevented by applying a generous coat of vaseline to susceptible areas. Treatment requires a stoppage of the physical activity and the application of an antiseptic lotion.

- Chondromalacia patella may be prevented by using an orthotic device in the shoes if needed, by reducing exposure to hard running surfaces, hills, and sloped terrains. Treatment includes rest, ice applications, and aspirin every four hours for a couple of weeks.

- Hamstring injuries may be prevented by daily stretching exercise. Treatment includes use of the RICE principle and stretching exercises.

- Prevention of low-back pain includes stretching the low-back muscles and the hamstring muscles and increasing the strength of the back and abdominal muscles. Treatment may include all of the above plus aspirin and a firm mattress.

- Prevention of Morton's neuroma includes wearing shoes that have a roomy toebox, are flexible, and well padded under the balls of the feet. Treatment includes the use of metatarsal bars under the ball of the foot, rest, and possible surgery.

- Prevention of muscle cramps includes stretching exercises and a gradual warm-up prior to exercise. Depletion of body fluids and minerals may also be involved. Treatment includes firm pressure at the site of the cramps. This should be followed by ice and stretching.

- Prevention of delayed muscle soreness includes exercising within one's capacity, by progressing slowly, by doing exercises, and by avoiding hilly terrain in the early stages of the exercise program. Treatment requires stretching and rest.

- Preventing plantar fasciitis involves well-fitted, well-cushioned walking and jogging shoes and stretching the calf and achilles tendon. Treatment consists of cold therapy, rest, anti-inflammatory drugs, heel pads, and possibly orthotic correction.

- Preventing shin splints includes wearing quality walking or jogging shoes, gradual adjustments in training, avoidance of hard surfaces and hilly terrain, proper heal-toe strike and stretching exercises. Treatment includes rest, ice, wrapping or taping the shin, and heel lifts in the shoes.

- Prevention of stress fractures means the avoidance of overuse. Too much exercise causes stress fractures. Treatment involves cutting back on mileage, stretching exercises, and walking or jogging on flat, softer surfaces.

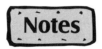

1. Hoeger, W. W. K. and Hoeger, Sharon A., *Lifetime Physical Fitness & Wellness: A Personalized Program* (Englewood, CO: Morton Publishing, 2000).

2. R. E. Leach et al., "Achilles Tendonitis," *Physician and Sportsmedicine*, 19 (Aug. 1991), 87.

3. T. P. White and Editors, University of California at Berkeley, Wellness Letter, *Wellness Guide to Lifelong Fitness* (Rebus, NJ: Random House, 1993).

4. D. J. Newham et al., "Large Delayed Plasma Creatine Kinase Changes After Stepping Exercise," *Muscle Nerve*, 6 (June 1983), 380.

5. D. S. Fick et al., "Relieving Painful Skin Splints," *Physician and Sportsmedicine*, 20:12 (Dec. 1992), 105.

6. R. D. Chadbourne, "A Hard Look at Running Surfaces," *Physician and Sportsmedicine*, 18:7 (July 1990), 102.

World Wide Website Resources

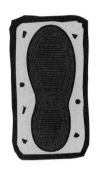

American Cancer Society
http://www.cancer.org/tobacco/index.html

American Diabetes Association
http://www.diabetes.org

American Dietetic Association
http://www.eatright.org

American Heart Association
http://www.americanheart.org

American Running Association
http://www.americanrunning.org/

Arizona Nicotine and Tobacco Network
http://www.tepp.org/

CNN's Health Report
http://www.cnn.com/HEALTH

Dr. Pribut's Running Injuries Page
http://www.clark.net/pub/pribut/spsport.html

Food and Nutrition Information Center
http://www.nal.usda.gov/fnic/

General Nutrition Site
http://www.healthy.net/index.html

Live Healthier Live Longer Cholesterol Counts for Everyone
http://rover.nhlbi.nih.gov/chd/

Mayo Clinic Health Information
http://www.mayo.ivi.com

National Osteoporosis Foundation
http://www.nof.org/

New Fitness
http://www.etonic.com/walking/fitness.html

Quantum Source Netsource for Exercise and Fitness Motivation
http://www.fitnessmotivation.com

Shape Up America!
http://www.shapeup.org/

Walking Wellness On-line
http://www.racewalk.com/WWBook/Ndefault.htm

Runner's World Training and Racing
http://www.runnersworld.com/training

Glossary

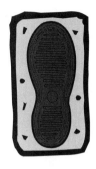

Adipose tissue   Fat cells in the body.

Aerobic   Literally meaning "with oxygen."

Aerobic capacity   Maximal amount of oxygen the human body is able to utilize per minute of physical activity (usually expressed in ml/kg/min).

Aerobic exercise   Activity that requires oxygen to produce the necessary energy to carry out the activity.

Allergen   Any substance that produces an allergic response.

Amino acids   Chemical compounds that contain nitrogen, carbon, hydrogen, and oxygen; the basic building blocks that the body uses to build different types of protein.

Amenorrhea   Cessation of the menstrual cycle.

Anabolism   The assimilation of nutrients and their conversion to living tissue.

Anaerobic   Literally meaning "without oxygen."

Anaerobic exercise   High-intensity activity that does not require oxygen to produce the desired energy.

Anaerobic threshold   The point during exercise at which blood lactate suddenly begins to increase.

Android obesity   Masculine pattern of body fat deposition in the abdomen, chest, and back.

Antioxidant   Compounds such as vitamins C, E, beta-carotene, and selenium that prevent oxygen from combining with other substances that it may damage.

Arterioles   Smallest arteries in the body.

Asthmogenic   Substances or events that are capable of producing bronchospasms.

Atherosclerosis   A slow, progressive disease of large and medium-size arteries characterized by the formation of plaque.

Atrophy   Decrease in the size of a cell.

Ballistic stretching   Exercises done with jerky, rapid, and bouncy movements.

Basal metabolic rate (BMR)   The minimum amount of energy the body expends to sustain life while at complete rest.

Blood plasma   The liquid portion of the blood.

Body composition   Proportionate amounts of fat and lean body tissues.

Body mass index (BMI)   Ratio of weight to height, used to determine thinness and fatness and risk for disease.

Carcinogenic   Describes substances that are capable of producing cancer.

Cardiac output (Q)   Represents the amount of blood pumped by the heart in 1 minute.

Cardiac reserve   The difference between HR max and RHR.

Cardiorespiratory endurance   Ability of the lungs, heart, and blood vessels to deliver adequate amounts of oxygen to the cells to meet the demands of prolonged physical activity.

Cardiovascular disease   Any illness of the heart and coronary blood vessels.

Catabolism   Breakdown of complex chemical compounds into simpler ones for use by the body.

Catecholamines   The hormones epinephrine and norepinephrine; stimulants to the circulatory system that constrict blood vessels.

Chronic diseases   Longlasting and/or frequently occurring illnesses.

Chronic stress   Long-term stress induced by persistent exposure to a stressor or group of stressors.

Clinical depression   Prolonged sadness that persists for some time without an identified cause (as in situational depression).

Communicable diseases   Diseases that can be transmitted from outside agents; also called infectious diseases.

Concentric muscle contraction   A reaction in which the muscle shortens while the individual lifts a weight against the force of gravity.

Conduction   Heat loss by physical contact between two objects.

Convection   Heat loss that occurs when a cooler gas or liquid flows across the skin.

Coronary heart disease (CHD)   Illness of the heart caused by atherosclerotic narrowing of the coronary arteries.

Cross-training   Training that utilizes a variety of activities rather than just one.

Dehydration   Excessive fluid loss from the body.

Degenerative disease   Chronic illness that becomes progressively worse over time.

Depression   Prolonged sadness that persists beyond a reasonable time.

Diastolic blood pressure   The pressure between heartbeats.

Distress   Negative stress.

Disuse atrophy   Premature loss resulting from under-stimulation.

Diuretic   Refers to substances that rid the body of excess water through urine.

DNA   Master blueprint for cellular function.

Duration   How long a person exercises.

Dynamic stretching   Stretching that involves bouncing and bobbing movements.

Eccentric muscle contraction   Lengthening a muscle while resisting the force of gravity as it returns to the starting position.

Electrocardiograph (ECG)   Measurement of electric activity of the heart.

Electrolytes   Ions that conduct electricity.

Essential fat   Body fat that is indispensable to normal physiological functioning.

Essential hypertension   Persistent high blood pressure that has no known cause.

Evaporation   The loss of body heat when liquid sweat is vaporized at the surface of the skin.

Exercise electrocardiogram (ECG)   An exercise test during which the workload is gradually increased (until the subject reaches maximal fatigue) with blood pressure and 12-lead electrocardiographic monitoring throughout the test.

Exercise heart rate   The heart rate that an exerciser needs to maintain to improve aerobic capacity.

Epinephrine   Hormone secreted by the adrenal glands that constricts blood vessels.

Estrogen   Female sex hormone thought to contribute to some disease conditions.

Eustress   Positive stress.

External (extrinsic) rewards   Reinforcement administered by outside sources.

Flexibility   Range of movement around joints of the body.

Folic acid   B vitamin that is necessary for controlling blood level of homocysteine.

Free radicals   Byproducts of oxidation that damage cells and DNA.

Frequency   Number of times per week a person participates in physical activity.

Goal   An end or objective to be achieved.

Gynoid obesity   The feminine pattern of body fat deposition in the hips, buttocks, and thighs.

HDL   High density lipoproteins, which scavenge cholesterol from tissues and bloodstream and transfer it back to the liver through intermediary carriers, for degradation, recycling, or disposal; "good cholesterol."

Health promotion   Fostering lifestyle behaviors conducive to health enhancement, such as exercise, smoking cessation, blood pressure screening, cholesterol evaluation, stress management, weight control.

Health-related fitness   Fitness goal that emphasizes development of cardiorespiratory endurance, muscular strength and endurance, flexibility, and lean body composition.

Heart rate reserve (HRR)   Difference between the maximal heart rate and the resting heart rate.

Hematocrit   Ratio of red blood cells to plasma volume.

Hemoglobin   Iron pigment of red blood cells that carries oxygen and carbon dioxide.

Homeostasis   State of equilibrium with respect to body functions and to the chemical composition of fluids and tissues.

Homocysteine   One of the amino-acid building blocks of protein; high levels damage arteries.

Hormone replacement therapy (HRT)   Replacing estrogen in the female usually after menopause, when its natural production stops.

Hydrogenated Hydrogen added to fats to increase shelf life and make the product more spreadable; increases saturation of the fat.

Hypertension Medical term for high blood pressure

Hyperthermia Excessive heat accumulation in the body.

Hypothermia Excessive heat lost from the body.

Inflammation Disease condition produced by infection, injury, or irritant, characterized by redness, swelling, and pain.

Insoluble fiber Dietary fiber in polysaccharides that is insoluble in hot water. It enhances the health of the intestines by speeding food remnants through them.

Insulin Hormone manufactured by the body that facilitates the passage of sugar from the blood to the cells.

Intensity Amount of energy expended per bout of exercise.

Internal (intrinsic) rewards Reinforcement coming from within the absence of some visible reward.

Ischemia Diminished blood flow to the heart.

Karvonen method One of the more accurate methods for determining exercise heart rate.

Kilocalories (kcals) Representing the number of calories found in food; also called calories.

Lactate threshold The point during exercise at which blood lactate suddenly begins to increase.

LDL Low density lipoproteins which transport cholesterol from liver to body cells; "bad cholesterol."

Lipids The scientific term for "fat."

Lipoproteins Carriers to which cholesterol attaches for transport through the circulatory system.

Lp(a) Lipoprotein (a) which in high levels can promote development of blood clots in the arteries.

Macronutrients One of two categories of minerals also known as major minerals.

Malignant Refers to tumors or tissues that are cancerous.

Maximal heart rate (MHR) Highest heart rate for a person, primarily related to age.

Menopause Decline and eventual cessation of hormone production by reproductive system in mid-life; termination of menstrual cycle.

Menstruation Monthly flow of blood from uterine lining; also termed *menses*.

Metabolic diseases Category of diseases involving body metabolism, including diabetes mellitus, thyroid disorders, kidney disease and liver disease.

Metabolism The sum of the chemical changes occurring in tissues consisting of anabolism and catabolism.

Micronutrients Trace minerals; nutrients in quantities less than 5 grams.

Morbidity Sick rate in a population.

Mortality Death rate in a population.

Motivation Internal mechanisms and external stimuli that arouse and stimulate behavior.

Muscular endurance Capacity to exert repetitive muscular force.

Muscular strength Maximum amount of force that a muscle or group of muscles can exert in a single contraction.

Myocardial infarction The medical term for a heart attack.

Myotatic reflex Response to forceful strength by a proprioceptor in the center of muscles.

Neoplasm New tissue or tumor.

Norepinephrine A hormone secreted by the adrenal glands that constricts blood vessels.

Nutrient density Ratio of nutrients to calories in food.

Nutrients Substances found in food that provide energy, regulate metabolism, and help with growth and repair of body tissues.

Obesity A chronic disease characterized by an excessively high amount of body fat in relation to lean body mass.

Oncogene A cancerous gene.

Orthotics Orthopedic devices placed in shoes to correct biomechanical problems.

Overfat Excessive fat: for males 23% to 25% or more of the body weight is fat and females 32% or more of the body weight is fat.

Overload Subjecting the various body systems to greater physical demand to produce muscle development.

Overtraining The onset of physiological and psychological staleness brought about by exclusive exercise.

Overweight Excessive body weight for height.

Oxidation The process that transforms food materials into heat or mechanical energy.

Oxygen debt The amount of O_2 required during recovery from exercise that is over and above that which is normally required at rest.

Oxygen deficit The first one or two minutes of exercise when the O_2 demand exceeds the body's ability to supply it.

Percent body fat Total amount of fat in the body based on the person's weight, includes both essential and storage fat.

Percent daily value The percentage of a food substance that is required on a daily basis.

Performance-related fitness The type of fitness that enables a person to perform physical skills with a high degree of proficiency.

Peripheral vascular resistance A body condition whereas the arterioles are in a constant state of slight contraction.

Peristalsis The waves of alternate contraction and relaxation that propel digested food along the colon.

Physical activity Bodily movement produced by skeletal muscles that requires energy expenditure and produces progressive health benefits.

Phytochemicals Compound found in fruits and vegetables that block the formation of cancerous tumors and disrupt the process.

Positive feedback reinforcement A reward or action that increases the strength of a response.

Progression Exposing body to greater and greater physical demands.

Proprioceptive neuromuscular facilitation (PNF) Stretching technique in which muscles are stretched out progressively with intermittent isometric contractions.

Radiation The loss of body heat through electromagnetic waves emitted to the environment.

Rate of perceived exertion (RPE) A perception scale to monitor or interpret the intensity of aerobic exercise.

Recommended dietary allowance (RDA) Daily suggested intakes of nutrients for normal, healthy people, as developed by the National Academy of Sciences.

Resting heart rate (RHR) Rate after a person has been sitting quietly for 15–20 minutes.

Resting metabolic rate (RMR) The amount of energy needed to sustain life in the rested but awake state.

RICE principle This is an acronym which stands for rest, ice, compression, and elevation of an injured body part.

Risk factors Genetic tendencies and learned behaviors that increase the probability of premature illness and death from specific diseases.

Self-motivation The desire to persist at a task without constant help or praise.

Serum cholesterol Cholesterol level in the blood.

Skinfold thickness Technique to assess body composition, including percent body fat, by measuring the thickness of skin at specified body sites.

Soluble fiber Dietary fiber that dissolves in hot water.

Specificity of training A principle stating that training must be done with the specific muscle the body is attempting to improve.

Static stretching Holding muscle positions in a fixed manner for 15 to 30 seconds.

Storage fat Body fat in excess of the essential fat; stored in adipose tissue.

Stressors Any condition, circumstance, or event that provokes the stress response.

Stroke volume The amount of blood the heart can eject in one beat.

Systolic blood pressure Represents the pressure of the blood against the artery walls when the heart contracts.

Target heart rate The heart rate that should be attained during aerobic exercise that will result in an improvement of aerobic capacity.

Thrombus A blood clot.

Transfatty acids Solidified fat formed by adding hydrogen to monosaturated and polyunsaturated fats to increase shelf life.

Triglycerides Fats formed by glycerol and three fatty acids.

Transtheoretical model for behavior change Behavioral theory characterized by stages of change.

Vasoconstriction Narrowing or clamping down of blood vessels.

Ventilation The amount of air moved in and out of the lungs in one minute.

VO$_2$ max Represents the body's peak ability to assimilate, deliver, and extract oxygen and is considered to be the best indicator of physical fitness.

Weight cycling Repeated weight loss and regain; also called yo-yo dieting.

Waist/hip ratio A test to assess potential risk for diseases based on body fat pattern distribution.

Index

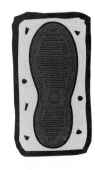